Dr Phil Hammond studied medicine (of sorts) at Cambridge University and St Thomas's Hospital, London. He qualified as a doctor in 1987. After house jobs in Bristol and Bath, he joined the Bath GP training scheme and in 1990 he formed the whistle-blowing double act *Struck Off and Die*, with Dr Tony Gardner. In five visits to the Edinburgh Festival they were twice selected for Perrier Pick of the Fringe and won Writers' Guild and Silver Sony awards for their first Radio 4 series. He has been medical correspondent for *Private Eye* since 1992 and repeatedly publicized the problems of child heart surgery in Bristol three years before anyone else. From 1996–1998 he was columnist for *The Independent* and he currently write for *The Express, Esquire* and *She*. In 1993, he was appointed Lecturer in General Practice at Birmingham Medical School and two years later he received the Owen Wade Award for teacher of the year.

Since 1996, Phil has been a Lecturer in Communication Skills at Bristol Medical School, and works part-time as a GP in Keynsham and is presenter of *Trust Me (I'm a Doctor)* (BBC2). In 1997 he was voted the Periodical Publications' Association Specialist Writer of the Year and in 1998 became Honorary President of the National Association of Non-Principals, an organization supporting GPs who are not in partnerships. He is married with two children and lives in Somerset.

Michael Mosley studied medicine at the Royal Free Hospital in London. After qualifying, he switched careers and took a job at the BBC as a trainee assistant producer. He has worked for the BBC for fourteen years, on current affairs programmes and in the Science Department. He has made a number of award-winning medical programmes and, in 1995, was named by the British Medical Association as their medical journalist of the year. He is currently the editor of *QED* as well as *Trust Me (I'm a Doctor)*, the first series of which won Gold and Silver Medals from the British Medical Association for excellence in medical broadcasting.

TRUST ME
(I'm a doctor)

Dr Phil Hammond
& Michael Mosley

metro

First published in Great Britain in 1999
by Metro Books (an imprint of Metro Publishing Limited),
19 Gerrard Street, London W1V 7LA

Phil Hammond and Michael Mosley are hereby identified as
the authors of this work in accordance with Section 77 of
the Copyright, Designs and Patents Act 1988.

British Library Cataloguing in Publication Data. A CIP
record of this book is available on request from the British
Library.

ISBN 1 900512 60 2

10 9 8 7 6 5 4 3 2 1

Typeset by Wakewing, High Wycombe, Buckinghamshire

Printed in Great Britain by CPD Group, Wales

CONTENTS

Introduction   vi

**Part One
Medical Culture – And What You Can Do
About It**

1. Medical School   3
2. Learning on the Job   22
3. Publish and Be Praised   44
4. Trust Me, I'm a Doctor   65
5. Help Me, I'm a Patient   87

**Part Two
A Consumer's Guide to Treatments**

6. You Are What You Eat   111
7. Life, Death and Vitamins   127
8. From Sperm to Baby   144
9. Common, Common, Common   166
10. The Alternatives   188
   Notes   200
   Index   205

INTRODUCTION

Why do you trust doctors? Because you want to, because you have to or because we deserve it? The late Dr Tom Chalmers, a champion of good medical research, once asked why doctors kill more people than airline pilots. He came up with ten reasons, such as pilots have to take time off for sleep, they are always under observation, they have to do everything in duplicate, they follow protocols, they have random breath testing and they have to be reassessed for their competency every six months. But he saved the best reason until last: 'If doctors died with their patients, they'd take a great deal more care.'

This book, and the BBC 2 series, *Trust Me (I'm a Doctor)*, on which it is based, is an attempt to give you an insider's guide to the practice of medicine and to the evidence that proves which commonly given treatments work and which don't. Medicine attracts a wide range of individuals, from dedicated altruists to self-deluded bodgers. We hope that by the time you've read this you'll be in a better position to find the former and avoid the latter. Most doctors try their best in difficult circumstances, but we need informed, assertive patients to ensure that this best is good enough. To participate in decisions about your health you need to be up to date on medical research (to find out the best thing to do), inquisitive about medical audit (to check that the best thing is being done) and numerate (to avoid ludicrous health scares). This book will help.

The first section of the book, Medical Culture – And What You Can Do About It, looks at the darker side of medicine and of medical training. You may or may not care that your doctor is particularly prone to alcoholism, depression and suicide, but these are the product of the pressures and destructive culture of medicine, which in turn affect the way your doctors treat you. Things are undoubtedly changing, but the changes are being driven more by the public exposure of gross failures than by any serious desire on the part of the medical establishment to reform itself. The scandal of the babies who died at Bristol Royal Infirmary is something that we've written about at length, partly because it's going to have a major impact on the future of medicine in this country, and partly because one of us was involved in the whole sorry tale, having been the first to break the news in *Private Eye* back in 1992.

To write the second section, A Consumer's Guide to Treatments, we have scoured the best medical journals in the world for studies which provide evidence for the effectiveness or otherwise of a range of common treatments. It's not exhaustive but should give useful, evidence-based information that is unlikely to change quickly. Most of the evidence we present is the result of many studies that have consistently said the same thing. This is important because in medical research studies frequently give conflicting results, so one study on its own proves nothing. They are not infallible but you are more likely to find good studies in the top medical journals, such as the *British Medical Journal*, the *Lancet, Journal of the American Medical Association*, and the *New England Journal of Medicine* than in most other publications. If you have access to the World Wide Web you may also want to look at some of the useful web sites we've used, namely:

American Medical Association:
    http://www.ama-assn.org/sci-pubs/pubsrch.htm
Bandolier: http://www.jr2.ox.ac.uk/Bandolier/
British Medical Association: http://www.bmj.com
The Lancet: http://www.lancet.com
Medline: http://www.ncbi.nlm.nih.gov/PubMed/
New England Journal of Med:
    http://www.nejm.org/content/index asp

Bandolier in particular is well worth a look because they do much of the hard work for you, pulling together as many good studies as they can and discarding the bad ones. We think it's wonderful.

Ultimately it is up to you to ask questions. It's certainly not easy challenging professionals and you may be tempted to lie back and take the path of least resistance. But there is good evidence that patients who become involved in their own healthcare do better and if you want a better health service you're going to have to do more than just pay for it, you're going to have to shape it. As *The Independent* critic Tom Sutcliffe observed of our TV series, 'A better title would be "Don't trust them just because they're doctors."'

Phil Hammond
Michael Mosley
January 1999

Part 1

MEDICAL CULTURE – AND WHAT YOU CAN DO ABOUT IT

1 | MEDICAL SCHOOL

"

'You say something like "I want to do something with science and care for people...or I just want to be a really ruthless bastard and not care for people."'

'As for your personal statement...even if you haven't done something write it down anyway. I put down that I'd done work experience but I didn't. I'd just be a cocky son of a bitch...'

Advice given by medical students to sixth formers attending University College London Medical School Open Day

Quotes taken from Making Doctors *(Berg, 1997) by doctor-turned-anthropologist Simon Sinclair who studied undergraduate medical training at University College London Hospital (UCLH) in 1993–4*

"

WHY DO YOU WANT TO BE A DOCTOR?

When I was seven my father, a senior lecturer in chemistry, locked himself in his lab and took his life. I write this not to shock, although the statistics for young male suicides are truly shocking, but by way of explanation. Had he not done so, I'd probably still be living in Australia and have had no contact at all with those two uniquely British white, male, middle-class dominated oligarchies, the National Health Service (NHS) and the BBC. As it was, we came back to live in England, I stayed white and male, became middle class and swapped nasal speech for Received Pronunciation. I did science A levels, partly in memory of my Dad, and when I did better than anticipated, I was expected to do medicine. Not by my Mum, who tried to get me to think through the consequences, but by my teachers. I didn't need much persuading; I'd seen *Doctor in the House* and I was in unrequited love for a girl who wanted to be a nurse.

There were other reasons too. My father had been an extremely gifted researcher and teacher, and wanted to use science for the good of humanity. So did I. Whether his death influenced my choice of career is hard to say. Some of us do choose medicine because of our own experience of illness or suffering, but I think I may have chosen it anyway.

With a family history of depression, I was perhaps unwise to choose the two professions (medicine and comedy) where the illness most prevails. Mercifully, the black dog hasn't bitten yet, but I wonder whether my unsubtle approach to demystifying medicine has something to do with wanting to change the system in case it does.

I was also influenced by my English teacher, Paddy O'Regan. In 1975, Marlborough Grammar School and Secondary Modern merged to form St John's Comprehensive and, as a result, the mixed-ability English class was born. For my sins, I used to snigger at the students with reading difficulties. Perhaps this was an early sign of the aggressive, competitive humour that so many doctors have. Anyway, Paddy spotted it and wrote on my report 'Philip might be bright but he would do well to consider those less fortunate than himself.'

He also believed in openness, and let his students read and criticize their reports before they were sent out. This is in marked contrast to medicine where, twenty-five years later, doctors still use secretive, closed references to stuff each other's careers. As it was, I read my report and had a tantrum. Paddy offered to rewrite it, but I grudgingly recognized the truth. It was the best piece of advice I've ever been given.

AN EXTENSION OF PUBLIC SCHOOL, ONLY WORSE

Three years later, I switched from comprehensive to public school to do my A levels. Boys who came late to the school were labelled 'anal entries' and I was also known (pejoratively rather than affectionately) as Phil From the Town. As nicknames went, it wasn't the worst; step forward Pubes Sweeting, Piggy Patterson, Bugger Ashley and Jock-Strap Jeans-Jacobson.

The language in general was mysteriously traditional (years were called shell, remove and hundreds, homework was called prep and teachers were called beaks) and there were very formal codes of conduct and discipline; students got blue chits and pink chits for stepping out of line, and only the prefects could walk on the grass.

Eight years on, in 1984, when I started clinical medicine in London, the similarities between medical school and public school were obvious.

The dean was head boy, the consultants were prefects and everyone else was a fag. The fags were finally free from the restraints of pink chits and lights out at 10.30p.m., and they went wild – but in a very conservative way. Paternalism and patronage were such that you didn't dare upset the establishment for fear of mucking up your reference; as a result, obsequious conformism and institutional loyalty ruled. Rebellious behaviour was either pharmacological escapism or aimed at the few things lower down the evolutionary ladder than you. These included patients, nurses, other students, bits of patients, bits of nurses or bits of each other's bodies – especially the bits in-between the femurs and slightly in front of the coccyx.

Language too had a traditional flavour. The course was 'pre-clin' or 'clin', and in clin we were assigned to firms with a Gauleiter. There was a school Beadle (called George), the parties were hops, the toilets were traps and trap number one belonged to The Syndicate. Use it at your peril. There was also a drinking club called The Clavicle, because of the number of students who had broken theirs after trying to drink a pint in twenty or so pubs in one evening. You had to wear evening dress for the attempt, but were allowed to vomit, urinate and fall over in public, provided you did so in a gentlemanly manner.

In private, anything went. The first day I walked into St Thomas's bar, I saw someone vomit on the dartboard from six feet. He's now a consultant orthopaedic surgeon. Another student was so desperate to win a game of Flaming A's, where two men are connected at the buttocks by a piece of burning lavatory paper, that he allowed the backs of his legs to be burnt. He's also an orthopaedic surgeon. At the Freshers' hop, one student urinated on a nurse claiming the dance was 'a gentleman's excuse me'. He's now a urologist.

Our japes were small fry compared to those of our predecessors, allegedly. There were stories of bladder tennis (where students catheterize each other, connect in the middle and try to pee into each other's bladders), freckle (where someone defecates on the table, hits it with a shoe and the person with the most freckles buys the next round) and bleep roulette. In this game, all the doctors on call put their bleeps into the middle of the table and select one at random. The surgeon on call ends up with the psychiatrist's bleep and vice versa.

Anyone who played rugby had a nickname. Mine was Fruithead, and I was put in charge of drinking games. If I asked Freshers to drink a pint of urine, vomit or even Heineken, they would, no questions asked. There was a strict hierarchy and everyone followed the rules.

The most important rule of all was 'what goes on tour, stays on tour.' You could do what you liked but you mustn't drop your mates in it when you got back. One year, we took a mutilated ox's head and assorted pots from the pathology museum (cancer of the vulva and cancer of the penis) on tour to Yorkshire, and used them as pub and touch line mascots. No one questioned this behaviour; it was as if we were somehow immune to what went on in the rest of society.

Like the Masons, of which there are a large number in medicine, we were bound by codes of loyalty and secrecy. Break them at your peril. On 7 September 1998, a letter was sent to me at *The Independent* saying 'Fruithead. We know who you are and we have the photos to prove it. Jobsworth.' I've no recollection who Jobsworth is (the postmark was Kingston upon Thames) but I'm sure he's got some disgusting photos of me as a student that will shortly be appearing in the tabloids.

This culture of secrecy permeates all levels of medicine, from the student bar to the reading room of the Royal College of Surgeons. God knows what Stinky, Shakey, Chopper and Smelly get up to in there, but none of the rest of us do. Lack of openness also means lack of accountability, or at least accountability left to the consciences of individual doctors and you wouldn't want to bet your life on that.

For those who played rugby, there was the unspoken promise that we would be looked after when it came to house-job applications. We were just the sort of bloody good chaps that make jolly good doctors. Although I committed myself to rugby at my interview (it was virtually the only question I was asked), I soon lost faith in treading on people in the name of sport and gave up. With this died my one chance of a teaching hospital job.

WHO GETS IN AND GETS ON

'I'm not having any fucking women in my department or any fucking Indians either. I just want to learn how to break the law.'

A hospital consultant at an 'equal opportunities' training session to encourage fairer job selection, November 1998

Fifty-three per cent of medical graduates are now women and although some are bullied and harassed, there is no evidence that they are discriminated against as students. In fact, at present your best chance of becoming a doctor is to be a 'white, middle-class, female, academic high achiever'.[1] However, there is a glass ceiling in many of the more macho specialities. In England, the number of female consultant surgeons has risen from 3 per cent in 1987 to only 5 per cent in 1997. In Scotland, the figure is even lower (4.2 per cent). I once met a female surgeon who was asked (illegally) at six consecutive consultant interviews, 'When are you going to have a baby?' She got so hacked off that before her seventh interview, she borrowed a uterus in a pot from her local pathology museum, put it in her handbag, took it along to the interview, plonked it on the desk and said 'Right, now let's talk about that job.' And she got it.

As for physicians, only 8.6 per cent of those in 'high-status' jobs – general medicine, cardiology, diabetes and endocrinology, gastroenterology, nephrology and thoracic medicine – are women. By contrast in 'low status' rheumatology (known as 'the housewife's speciality'), 16.2 per cent of consultants are women and in 'unscientific and ineffective' psychiatry the figure is 29.8 per cent. The one high-status speciality where women have broken through is paediatrics where 33.6 per cent of consultants are women, presumably because they're 'good with children'.

If you're not white, things are rather tougher. The *BMJ* research (24/10/98) found that eighteen out of twenty-seven medical schools 'disadvantaged' applicants from ethnic minority groups. As Manchester GP and researcher Aneez Esmail put it: 'Some deans have privately said there are "too many" Asians in medical schools.' Those from working-class backgrounds were also less likely to succeed.

In the 1930s, the good doctors of Guy's Hospital in London used to make up for the lack of black faces by darkening up, referring to each other as 'Massa' and appearing as a jolly singing troupe, the Christmas Niggers. Here's an extract from Guy's Hospital *Gazette*:[2]

> The group of coloured gentlemen gathered before a camera on the steps of the Colonnade on the morning of Christmas Day were not, as we heard an old lady suppose, distinguished visitors being introduced to the hospital by its chaplains. It is true, however, that in a sense they were missionaries. They were, in fact (reader, you have guessed it already), the 'Niggers' performing their annual mirth mission.

In the thirties every hospital may have had a sub-Minstrels singing troupe but it's not something you'd generally want to draw attention to. Nearly fifty years later, Guy's *Gazette* ran a double-page celebration of The Niggers. The same hospital was also pilloried in the House of Commons for including racist jokes in its rag mag; its defence was that one of the students on the rag committee was Asian and he didn't mind.

At St Thomas's in 1986 the influx of very bright Asian students caused grief to some. As one consultant put it: 'I've got nothing against them *per se*, but most of them don't drink or play rugby, and even if they did they wouldn't be much good. You can't push in the scrum if you're fasting for Ramadan.'

So, what happens to Asian medical students? In 1992 Drs Sam Everington and Aneez Esmail decided to find out. They sent fake applications to junior hospital doctor posts, identical in all but surname. Half the names they used were Asian, half were Anglo-Saxon. The latter were twice as likely to be offered an interview.

When this was published in 1993[3] the response of the medical establishment was swift and extraordinary. The racism was not admitted and investigated; instead, the pair were reported to the police, arrested and charged with fraud by the good folk at Hendon police station. The charge was quickly dropped but the General Medical Council (GMC) unwisely suggested the research was unprofessional. This infuriated the pair so much that they decided to investigate the GMC's disciplinary procedures. They discovered that the GMC was much more likely to discipline an ethnic minority doctor than a white doctor. This was not, however, due to a persecution of ethnic minority doctors. Rather it suggested that white doctors are far more likely to get away with misconduct.[4]

Everington and Esmail were motivated to undertake their covert research by the experience of Dr Mohammed Ashraf Memon, a junior surgeon so dedicated that he passed the Fellowship of the Royal College of Surgeons three times, in Dublin, Edinburgh and London. Many would say this was needless duplication, yet ethnic minority doctors consistently have to prove their excellence and dedication. Despite his qualifications, Dr Memon was unable to secure a post at Bart's Hospital and subsequently won a settlement for discrimination at an industrial tribunal. Not that it did his career any good. He was subsequently blacklisted and his career came to a halt. Dr Memon has since moved to the United States.

In 1997, Everington and Esmail published a repeat experiment of their bogus application study for senior house officer posts in a variety of hospital specialities and GP training schemes.[5] Despite the passage of five years and many assurances from the profession's leaders that racism was being stamped out, little had changed. Thirty-six per cent of the Asian candidates were short listed, compared to 52 per cent of the Caucasians. And for those who do manage to get in and get on, ethnic minority doctors are three times less likely to end up with a lucrative merit award.[6]

DISSECTION

I started at Cambridge University in 1981 and the first patient I met was a dead one. Without any attempt at moral guidance, we were encouraged to cut our body up into increasingly smaller pieces, roughly in line with the text book. Some students fainted, a few juggled with the kidneys or skipped with the intestines. I practised spin-passing with a heart. One amusing man stuck a hose in one end of the gut and blasted the contents out of the other. How we all laughed.

Then there were apocryphal stories of bits that had been smuggled out. A student was said to have stolen an arm and hidden it at the bottom of his girlfriend's bed. Others favoured an aberrant penis, on a key ring or dropped between tube doors or in a rugby scrum. No one ever did it but we talked about it a lot.

Not all students exhibited such disregard for human death. The pair dissecting opposite me were scholars. They took it all very seriously and meticulously dissected out every tiny root of the autonomic nervous system running alongside the spine. It must have taken hours and was truly a beauty to behold...until Jocky, my dissection partner mistook it for fat and ripped the whole lot out. It was the only time I ever saw anyone cry in the dissection room – but then I wasn't there when a student pulled back his sheet and allegedly discovered a cadaverous Auntie Beryl.

Human dissection was a rite of passage, the one thing that separated us from other students. It started in Britain in the sixteenth century using the bodies of criminals executed for murder. Being cut up by a medical student was seen as a further punishment, worse than gibbeting, and volunteers were thin on the ground. So doctors looked under it. Raiding paupers' graves to obtain 'resurrected corpses' was endemic in the eighteenth century – two thousand snatches a year for medical schools until the Anatomy Act tried to stop it in 1832. Dissection, however, carried on apace using 'unclaimed bodies'. Of the 57,000 cadavers used in London medical schools until the 1930s, virtually all were from workhouses or asylums – people who never consented to be dissected but had no one willing or able to afford a coffin.

I had no preparation for what lay behind the dissection room door – the God-awful smell, the sound of the saw slicing off the top of the skull or the sight of unfeasibly large genitals swollen in the preservation process. It was sink or swim, survival of the cruellest. In his book *Making Doctors*, Sinclair found a student who dreamt of eating the flesh she was dissecting. Another thought that this would be 'a fantastic possibility.'

I didn't think that deeply about it. Indeed, the only reference to the grisly business came in an aside in a pathology lecture: 'One man wanted to be a doctor but repeatedly failed his exams. When he died, he left us his body because it was the only way he'd ever get into medical school.' It was meant as a joke, but it inadvertently reminded us that this poor sod had never achieved his aspirations and was trying to do us a favour in death. How would he feel about our *laissez faire* attitude to his dismembered remains? My juggling stopped soon after.

Nowadays, students get introductory lectures on the ethics of cadaver use and a chance to discuss their feelings about meeting their first corpse. Only a few schools still let students do a lot of dissection unsupervized. Instead of getting a scalpel, a DIY guide book and half a body each, most students get to watch someone else do it properly from a distance. Any kidney juggling is done with plastic replicas.

SECRET LANGUAGE

At the start of my course I was told I would learn more new words in two years than a student of Russian. I doubt this was true, but there was certainly a lot of schoolboy Greek about and none of it made much sense. Could you discuss the aetiology, pathogenesis and epidemiology of menorrhagia? The latter comes from 'Men' (month) and 'rhegynai' (to rush out) – heavy periods. For menstruation alone, there's also dysmenorrhoea (painful periods), oligomenorrhoea (infrequent periods), amenorrhoea (absent periods) and polymenometrorrhagia (frequent, heavy, irregular periods). Travel an inch or so upwards and you can have dysuria (painful weeing), haematuria (bloody wee) and polyuria (lots of wee).

The charitable view of medspeak is that it allows doctors to communicate with each other effectively and quickly; for instance, 'Mrs

Simpson is oriented times three, PERLA, cranials II to XII intact, LFs clear, JVP not displaced, Heart Sounds I plus II plus nil, Abdo NAD, TPCSR in RUL equals LUL equals RLL equals LLL.' All it really means is that Mrs Simpson is judged fit to be turned out into the community but if you can say it with a straight face and you know where the hospital laundry is, you can impersonate a doctor for life.

Patients, being generally frightened and in awe, tend not to ask for an interpreter when doctors lapse into jargon, with predictable consequences. A study of 100 patients interviewed within five days of major abdominal surgery found that twenty-seven didn't know which organ had been removed and forty-four were unaware of the exact nature of the surgical procedure, despite having been counselled before the operation.[7]

Of course we wouldn't get away with it without the complicity of patients. There's a basic human need for magic and as scientific medicine is endlessly demystified in the media, people are flocking back to complementary therapies. 'I've got too much jitsu in my tsubo, you say? That'll do nicely – here's £50'. Also, there are a fair few people out there who enjoy being sick and for them a fancy diagnosis is essential. 'You've got a supracapsular bursitis' is much more impressive sounding than 'You've got a sore shoulder.'

TRAINING

A key feature of the old-style apprenticeship in clinical medicine was students trudging around teaching hospitals in the wake of great men, hoping to pick things up on the way. Sometimes you waited hours for the great man to arrive. When he did turn up he walked straight past you because he didn't have the faintest idea what you looked like. It was all very unsatisfactory, but at least you had access to patients.

When I moved to St Thomas's I met lots of them, sometimes in a 'let's all stare at you from the end of the bed' situation, occasionally in a 'let's all examine you under anaesthetic and hope you don't notice' situation, but mostly awake and in private, or at least as much privacy as a pair of NHS curtains would allow. Despite the two-foot gap for the voyeur in the bed opposite, the patients I met were unbelievably tolerant and helpful. Some even seemed pleased to be practised on by students who knew all about the Citric Acid Cycle but had never been taught to listen.

However, it was never very clear what we were supposed to be learning. The curriculum wasn't defined, there were no aims and objectives, no audit and no quality control. You just learned to examine whatever body system your consultant specialized in. Or you taught yourself if he wasn't there and bought a textbook, preferably the one written by your consultant. If you could regurgitate that, you were generally home and dry. No one pointed out that some of the information in a textbook is out of date by the time it hits the shelf, and we didn't learn how to analyse the studies on which the text was based. After three years of rote learning, we forgot how to think and ended up demanding spoon-feeding. As a patient, you can stop most doctors in their tracks by asking them to quote the evidence on which their treatment proposals are based. Be prepared for a lot of hedging in the answer.

SECRECY AND TRUTH TELLING

Perhaps the key attitude preventing doctors from being good, rather than barely adequate, was the belief that patients needed to be protected from the truth. As the American physician Oliver Wendell Holmes put it in a graduation speech to students in 1871: 'Your patient has no more right to all the truth you know than he has to all the medicine in your saddlebags… He should get only so much as is good for him.'

For another century, doctor–patient communication was a one way process. Doctor talked, patient listened, patient didn't understand a word but felt too in awe to say anything, consultation ended with pink medicine. Or sometimes abuse. Eric Cassell, a prominent physician in the 1930s, once accompanied his grandmother to see a specialist about a melanoma on her face. 'During the course of the visit when she asked him a question, he slapped her face saying, "I'll ask the questions here, I'll do the talking."'

In the early 1980s, a survey of British GPs and hospital consultants found that 75 per cent and 56 per cent, respectively, kept cancer patients in the dark.[8] In 1984, I was taught by a consultant who used to skirt around cancer with cricketing analogies. Patients were 'batting on a bit of a sticky wicket' or 'going to join the club-house in the sky.' And in 1993, 60 per cent of European gastroenterologists kept mum about cancer.[9] It was assumed that the patients would get upset and didn't really want to know. The truth might even kill them.

In 1996, a Scottish study discovered a different view. Of 250 patients attending a cancer centre, 96 per cent specifically wanted to know if their illness was cancer and 79 per cent wanted as much information as possible. Almost all wanted to know the chance of cure and the side effects of treatment.[10] That same year, I started teaching communication skills at Birmingham medical school and the students told me of a consultant who routinely said to cancer patients 'Your cells have been a little bit naughty.' Others had 'a tiny spot on the liver', 'a warty growth' or 'a bit of a problem down below.'

Thankfully, the majority of students and doctors I've worked with have been honest and compassionate communicators. However, there are still great chunks of information that are kept from patients. NHS staff are so squeezed for time that an increasing reliance is placed on leaflets and videos. In 1998 Angela Coulter of the King's Fund reviewed thousands of these and found that 'far too many of them adopt the paternalistic view that patients cannot cope with bad news and must be kept ignorant of medical uncertainties. Patients are seen as children in need of instruction and reassurance rather than experts in their own needs and preferences.'

Doctors, like everyone else, have a need to justify what they're doing. Hence 'benefits of interventions are emphasized, risks and side effects glossed over and scientific controversies hardly ever mentioned. In too many cases, the information contained in patient information leaflets is inaccurate or misleading.' If you want accurate, balanced, in-depth information, check out the latest research and don't count on doctors to provide all the answers.

BRUTALIZATION AND FEEDBACK

Of course, not all patients want to know the truth and even today doctors seek to protect certain groups of patients, such as those with dementia, from reality.[11]

The trend has now shifted towards openness about the diagnosis, if not the limits of the treatment, but there are still worries about the manner in which this information is given. Brutal honesty can be as damaging as hiding the truth. An ear, nose and throat surgeon in London says to patients, 'You know what your problem is, don't you? You've got cancer and you're going to die.' When I taught in a hospice, I noticed that the patients there had a very clear memory of how the bad news was first broken to them; it had a profound effect on the grieving process and how they coped psychologically. If it's done well, you never forget. If it's done badly, you never forgive.

It is as important for doctors to acquire communication skills as resuscitation skills, but I had to wait until I'd been qualified for seven years before I received any training in this area. And yet at medical school, a lot of the humour revolved around doctors who had allegedly said crass and insensitive things to patients. For instance, 'I'm not entirely sure what the diagnosis is – but I'm sure we'll find out at the post mortem' or 'I've got some good news and some bad news for you. The bad news is that one of us has got cancer. And the good news is, it's not me.' I once sat in on a gynaecology clinic when the doctor said, 'Well my dear, you'll be pleased to know you don't have cervical cancer... Oh yes, you do! My mistake. I was reading the wrong page.'

Empathy is a big problem for some medical students. I heard of one who stripped a patient and examined him, completely naked, without drawing the curtains. When a nurse marched up to demand what was happening, he said, 'It's OK sister, he's blind.' Another got so engrossed in reading off a long list of important questions that he failed to realize his patient was deaf. He'd been writing down the answers from a blind patient in the next bed.

Students are supposed to learn from their consultants, but some are less than ideal role models, as this student describes: 'We were on a ward round with a consultant paediatrician, and he burst into a room without knocking where two parents were sitting on the bed, cradling a Down's syndrome baby. Without acknowledging them at all, he turned to us and said, "Got the diagnosis?" – and then left the room.'

Today all medical students are obliged to receive communication skills training but it is received with varying degrees of enthusiasm and success. I'm fortunate enough to teach students using a talented team of simulated patients. These are actors who take on roles as patients and offer constructive feedback, allowing the students to practise and gain competence in such skills as breaking bad news, managing complaints, relating to relatives and explaining complicated treatments.

The courses are enthusiastically received by junior students, but as they get older the cynicism of medicine starts to kick in and they have to be coaxed into improving these vital skills. This observation is not unusual – studies have shown that students entering medical school are usually more idealistic and enthusiastic, and better communicators, than those leaving it. The GMC has done much to define the content of the course but medical culture is proving much harder to change.

BULLYING, COMPLAINING AND WHISTLE-BLOWING

Medicine has traditionally been a macho apprenticeship based on teaching by humiliation. Professor Chris Bulstrode, an orthopaedic surgeon turned medical teacher, recalls his first operation as a senior house officer working at the London hospital in 1974:

> An elderly woman came in with a fractured neck of femur (broken hip) who needed emergency surgery. I didn't have a clue how to do it, so I phoned my senior registrar for help. He was in Kent. I explained that I'd never done an operation before, he swore for ten minutes and after much argument agreed to come in. An hour later, he burst into the operating theatre, still in his suit, put some gloves on, made his incision, pinned and plated the broken hip, dropped his gloves on the floor and said, in front of all the theatre staff, 'Don't you ever call me at home again.' It was the most humiliating experience of my life.

Professor Bulstrode had to rely entirely on a theatre nurse to show him how to stitch the patient back up again. Subsequently, she taught him basic skills in other operations and he says, 'Without her, I'd have just given up.' After this experience, he vowed to make medical training more structured and humane. His training courses for surgeons have been a huge success, although, again, changing the culture has been an uphill struggle.

In 1995, when I was lecturing in Birmingham, a female student described assisting a surgeon at a laparoscopic cholecystectomy (removal of the gallbladder):

> First he asked me if I was from the Home Counties. When I said yes, he started calling me Tinkerbelle and said I looked the sort of girl who'd had a horse between my legs. Then he asked me if I'd lost my virginity up against the wall of a horse-box while my mother was outside watching a gymkhana. The registrar and the other theatre staff started laughing too. It was like being in a monkey house. At the end, he asked me if I minded him being sexist in theatre – 'Women like to know what men want'. Then he made a hole in the gall-bladder and said, 'Look what you've made me do.'

Most students are too frightened to complain, but I have known a female student extract a written apology from a professor of surgery after he tried the common bullying technique of insisting she examine a man's genitals in front of everyone on a packed ward round. 'You must have felt testicles before. Haven't you got a boyfriend?'

Another student told me a story which I suspect, or hope, is apocryphal. A student was on a gynaecology attachment to a district general hospital. He was a rugby player and a drinker, but like many of that ilk was deeply respectful of medical authority and frightened of consultant surgeons. The surgeon he was attached to is noted for his ferocity so the night before starting, the student – whom we shall call Toby – consoled his nerves with curry and lager.

The following morning, he assisted the surgeon in performing a vaginal hysterectomy. The advantage of this approach is that you can remove the womb without leaving a scar. Towards the end of a successful operation, Toby's curry and nerves got the better of him and he flatulated quietly but noxiously. The consultant sniffed the air, turned to his registrar and said, 'I smell faeces'. 'So do I,' sniffed the registrar. 'Damn,' said the consultant, 'We must have perforated the bowel.'

Toby considered the situation. Perforation of the bowel is a serious, often fatal, condition. If you suspect it, you have to reach for the scalpel and open up the abdomen. Did he own up and risk the surgeon's wrath and a bad reference? Or did he keep silent and watch a woman have an unnecessary bowel exploration, a large scar and all the pain and inconvenience it entails? He stayed silent.

True or not, I use this as an ethical dilemma for my students, together with the question 'What would you do if you found your consultant pissed in the car park?' They all find it amusing but the good news is that they are all patient-centred (at least publicly) and would risk their own reference for the sake of an anaesthetized woman. The only exception was a student who decided the way out was to lean forward and whisper to the consultant, 'I think it was sister.' That's another enduring medical attitude. If in doubt, blame it on the nurses.

Just Practising

I first began to doubt the wisdom of medicine when a professor of pathology told me: 'At post-mortem, half of what's written on the death certificate turns out to be wrong.' Were doctors really that bad at getting the diagnosis right? He also pointed out that, for many of the patients who died during or shortly after an operation, post mortem wasn't often requested. Even when it was, it revealed that many patients were too sick to stand any chance of surviving surgery. Could it really be that frail, elderly patients were being used as midnight cannon fodder for unsupervised trainees? He told me that when doctors go on strike, the death rate actually goes down.

This thought came home to roost in my final year when I nearly killed a patient. I was invited to do a locum for a house officer on holiday and, not wanting to let on that I didn't think I was up to it, I accepted. I could just about take blood, but had never been shown how to put up a drip. I bluffed my way through a night on call until, at five in the morning, I was called to re-site a drip.

The more senior doctors were in bed and I was too frightened to wake anyone. So I experimented with the drip and, thinking I'd got it in the vein, flushed it through with saline. The patient screamed and complained of pain in her hand. I'd injected potassium, which came in an identical bottle to the saline; at five in the morning in a dim light it was an easy mistake to make. Had the drip been properly in the vein, the patient would have had a cardiac arrest. Fortunately, it wasn't and she suffered a swollen, painful hand instead. I apologized and lied, telling her she must be allergic to saline. I felt awful, told a friend and guess what? It appeared in the student magazine.

My experience was not unusual. Another student 'acted up' for a house officer who was off sick on an attachment to a district hospital. On his first day, the hospital was so busy that he was left alone with a man who had an aneurysm (swelling) of his aorta (the biggest artery in the body). It burst in front of him and he desperately tried to resuscitate the patient, putting drips in both arms, successfully, getting fluid in, cross matching blood and calling for help. It took a long time coming and, just as he thought he'd done everything, the man vomited, aspirated into his lungs and died. The student had forgotten to put an airway in. Hardly surprising since no one had ever even told him to, let alone showed him how. This is how bad medical training could be, and still can. The doctor, now a GP, is still very affected by what happened.

STRESS AND ALCOHOL

There is a great fear amongst medics of being seen not to cope or becoming patients. So we cope with drugs and inappropriate laughter. In two studies printed in the *Lancet*, researchers found that not only were heavy drinking and illicit drug use common amongst second year students, but also they increased after qualifying.[12, 13] Of the ninety house officers studied, 60 per cent of both sexes exceeded their safe limits. Thirty-five per cent of men and 19 per cent of women were using cannabis and 13 per cent of men and 10 per cent of women reported using other drugs such as hallucinogenic mushrooms, LSD, ecstasy, amyl nitrite, cocaine and amphetamines.

As for their mental state, 21 per cent of men and 45 per cent of women had anxiety scores indicating possible pathological anxiety. Clearly medical school is not only very stressful, but also does little to prepare students for the stresses of being a house officer. Still, you can always laugh it off.

GOOD HUMOUR?

A lot of advertisements for partners in general practice say 'good sense of humour essential', but never define what they mean by 'good'. The spoof Freshers' lecture is still alive and kicking in medicine, years after it died out in other disciplines. A commonly used format is to introduce a mature student as a lecturer in genito-urinary medicine. He, and it usually is a he, delivers an entirely credible lecture with gut-churningly credible slides on sexually transmitted diseases. Afterwards, he announces that he's conducting research into the sexual habits of medical students and asks for their help in a show of hands. He also insists that every student closes his or her eyes to ensure the answers remain strictly confidential.

He then asks the students to raise their hands to correspond with the number of sexual partners they've had, asking, 'Who's never had a sexual partner? Who's only ever had one? Who's had more than one?' and so on. Amazingly, the majority of students conform and with their eyes closed don't realize that whenever they raise their hands, their photographs are being taken for distribution around the medical school. In one school, they put up a special notice board for the virgins, with students crossed off as they lose the label.

Whether anyone minds is hard to judge, as no one must be seen to mind. As a GP told me last year: 'I still have vivid memories of our spoof lecture. I was sitting at the back next to a large woman and all of a sudden, the lights went down, they turned a spotlight on her and said, "Come on down, you fat slag." I laughed with everyone else but I just thought, thank Christ she's fatter than I am.' And a female student in her final year at Birmingham told me about her first experience in the medics' bar. 'A boy walked up and, without asking, put his penis in my pint.' She never went in there again.

Letting women in has done little to change the culture, and I get the feeling that many students don't actually want it to change. Some even seem to enjoy humiliation. If ever I needed proof, it was attending the Final Year Dinners (FYDs) at Birmingham Medical School between 1994 and 1996. When I'd taught the students, they were mainly bright, switched on and compassionate. But out of hours, they really laid into each other.

At the first FYD I went to, awards had to be collected for 'Slag of the Year' and 'Ugliest Person in the Year'. By the time I left, these had at least been refined to 'Smut Monkey of the Year' and 'Person Likely to have the Ugliest Children'. There were awards for half the year, ranging from 'Person of the Opposite Sex You Would Most Like to Catheterize' to 'Person Most Likely to Have ECT for Intractable Depression' and 'First into De-Tox'. There was a 'Dresses Like a Grandmother' award, a 'Singularly the Most Irritating Christian in the Year' award and a 'Biggest Politically Correct Tits Ever' award.

Not everyone found it funny (the Slag of the Year burst into tears as she accepted her commemorative T-shirt) but on the whole, it was seen as an OK thing to do because everyone was involved. If you didn't get an award, you copped it elsewhere. One confused male student foolishly asked his housemate for advice: 'What's that second hole in the end of your penis for? You know, there's one that you pee out of but what's the other one for?' Whether he got the urology referral he needed is unclear, but he got pride of place in the yearbook.

I'm sure the presence of more women in medical schools has put a curb on the worst excesses of male student behaviour, but it has certainly not stopped it. In 1996, we tried to interview some students at a London teaching hospital about their drinking habits. A few years previously, the Freshers had been subjected to a 'drink your way around the world' competition where they had to down a measure of spirits from every country and several ended up in casualty.

However, in 1996, the cameras weren't allowed in because some of the Freshers had been taken on tour and had been encouraged to drink Bloody Marys made out of their own blood, extracted using drip needles. The doctor in charge was disciplined not for encouraging the act itself, but for misappropriating NHS resources to extract the blood.

In the mid-1980s, AIDS arrived and medical revues had a field day. The year before I started at St Thomas's, the drama club rejigged Village People's YMCA to AIDS, with the words: 'Young man, You won't live to be old, I said, Young man, you'd better not catch a cold' etc. This was at a time when HIV-positive patients were being greeted by porters in 'high-risk space suits' and treated with widespread prejudice.

Humour is also used in medicine to disguise the inadequacy of the training. Very few students have a chance to discuss, reflect and come to terms with difficult but common dilemmas such as how to behave with a patient they find sexually attractive. No one is going to actually admit to sexually assaulting patients but a student wrote in the *Student BMJ* about a close call:

> A 19-year-old woman was admitted to hospital for cystoscopy to investigate the possible causes of urinary tract infections. I immediately noticed that she was very attractive. I began clerking but got nowhere, as I found myself staring into a pair of inviting blue eyes. The patient appeared to have developed an affection for me. As I plugged away with totally inane questions, I realized how devious I could be. I ran through a list of differential diagnoses trying to find one that would require me to examine her ample breasts that were being shoved towards me...

The student didn't succumb to the temptation, at least not that he admitted in print, but he felt guilty for even having the thought ('you probably think I'm a worthless lump of hormone'). However, other doctors I've spoken to have admitted to it. As one put it: 'I wouldn't do a TUBE [totally unnecessary breast examination] as a consultant, but as a student it was seen as a perk of the job.'

ASSESSMENT

Just as there was no clearly defined moral code or curriculum with aims and objectives for me to follow as a student, the assessment process was equally unreliable. Worst were 'firm grades', seemingly random allocations given by consultants who had no recollection of you, and whose marks often bore no relation to attendance or ability. Multiple choice questions were used to check if any 'facts' had been picked up and, although reliable, there was no test of whether these facts could be used appropriately in a clinical situation. The clinical exams consisted of short and long cases, followed by vivas. No one observed me interact with a patient. There was no evidence of objectivity, no structured marking schedule and great scope for unfairness.

Most students got through, possibly not on merit but because of the tacit assumption that a lot of failures would reflect badly on the teaching standards in the medical school. There was no public guarantee that this shambolic process produced students who were fit to progress to house officers and no evidence that we had the necessary skills. I left medical school without being sure I could measure blood pressure properly, without being able to put in a drip or a catheter, and with no idea how to break bad news or manage the sick patients I was about to be confronted with. I didn't learn to resuscitate a patient until long after I'd started carrying the emergency bleep.

Some medical schools have now made great strides towards making student assessment fairer and more objective, and testing that students have the basic skills to become house officers. As with the quality of the teaching – ironically often worst in teaching hospitals – this process is decidedly patchy and there is still a tendency to shepherd students through even if they haven't learnt a key skill. The comment, 'His blood pressure measurement was hopeless but the resuscitation wasn't bad so we'll pass him' is not untypical.

There is still a worry that if student assessment is rigorous, as it surely should be given the millions of pounds of public money poured into medical schools and the responsibilities of those leaving them, the number of failures will expose the paucity of the teaching. Some doctors claim that they are too busy fulfilling their NHS duties to teach and besides, most have never received any teacher training. But a teaching hospital receives a large sum of taxpayers' money – typically £6 million a year – to do just that, so there is no excuse. Much of the money, however, is used on patients and to prop up the NHS. Students are left to pick things up as they go along and when they qualify, they face the steepest learning curve of their life. August 1, when the new doctors turn out, is known as the Killing Season.

2|LEARNING ON THE JOB

'There was a lack of adequate supervision for junior doctors. I found the "see one, do one, teach one" mentality horrifying.'

'Long hours, unfair responsibilities, little supervision or encouragement that was constructive.'

Two junior doctors explain why they gave up medicine. From Don't Waste Doctors *(September 1998), a study commissioned by the North-west region to discover why 32 per cent of senior house officer posts were unfilled.*

'I see thirty patients in a three-hour clinic. I only have time to see them as walking tumours.'

A consultant oncologist

HOUSE JOBS

Given the quality of undergraduate medical training, it is surprising how many students progress to become dedicated and compassionate doctors. But not all.

In 1997, 8 per cent of medical graduates left the profession without completing their first year as a house officer and recent research suggests that an increasing number of UK graduates are not committed to practising medicine in the UK.[1] At up to £250,000 a time for their training, this is an expensive loss. It's clearly not only the fault of medical schools, which are trying to improve. Some parts of the NHS are just deeply unpleasant to work in. One student I taught who had excellent communication skills started a tough house job and received her first complaint in the first week. Having put in eighty hours, she was asked by the patient if there was any guarantee that his treatment would work. She lost her self control temporarily and snapped, 'If you want a guarantee, buy a toaster.'

My house jobs were comparatively humane. The best thing St Thomas's ever did for me was to give me a bad reference, namely, 'This student refuses to take medicine seriously and does not deserve a St Thomas's house job.' I was, of course, not told what my reference said. Instead I went from interview to interview wondering what I was doing wrong until, after five failures, I was rescued by a cardiologist and a surgeon in two friendly West-country district general hospitals. I was hopelessly unprepared for either job and relied almost exclusively on the nurses to show me what to do. They taught me more about being a doctor in two weeks than I'd picked up in six years at medical school.

In 1988, as a house-officer in Bath, I had my first hint that all was not well with cardiac surgery in Bristol. I was asked to go with a patient in an ambulance to Southampton. It was thought that the patient might have a tear in his aorta, an artery that comes out of the heart. Bath did not do heart surgery but Bristol and Southampton did. When I asked why the patient could not go to Bristol, which was much nearer, I was told, 'We don't refer to Bristol.' 'Why not?' 'We just don't.'

I was later told that not only was there an acrimonious regional dispute between the hospitals but also there were doubts about the ability of one of the surgeons there, whose nickname was 'Killer'. This was neither Mr Wisheart nor Mr Dhasmana, later investigated by the GMC, both of whom were considered extremely dedicated and capable.

Surgeons occasionally pick up nicknames such as 'Chopper' or 'Slasher' or 'Hacker', but without hard evidence you can't say whether these titles are macho terms of endearment or reflect a terrible reality. Gynaecologist Rodney Leward, struck off by the General Medical Council in September 1998, was nicknamed 'The Butcher' by his colleagues. Unfortunately they didn't report his incompetence to the GMC and he practised as a consultant for sixteen years before he was stopped, leaving behind many victims of his botched surgery. The women he treated were too embarrassed or in awe to complain, and the secretive and largely non-existent 'self-regulation' of the medical profession gave them no protection at all. If you don't know the competence of your local consultant surgeon, then your best chance may be to sneak into the next hospital revue – there's sure to be a sketch about him.

As for the patient with the torn aorta, we had a petrifying 90-minute drive to Southampton, with me not knowing what I would do if the heart burst on the way and him sensing I didn't. We both survived, but it was a situation that was completely beyond my competence. In 1991, a study published interviews with doctors in the South-west region carried out in the year after they qualified, hammering home the stress they feel and the effect this has on patients:[2]

When things are not going well you get blamed for almost every mistake. That kind of day makes you want to get out of the hospital as quickly as you can. So you might cut corners. If you're irritated and angry, it is going to come across to the patient and if you're busy as well you give them less time. Patients are often nervous and anxious and you really need to reassure them but you find you are being curt with them instead.

The main thing here is being so fed up. Nobody cares about you. Its not just the sleep, you can't get food at night, you spend ages trying to find ECG machines... It goes on and on. And the one thing you don't do when you're fed up is go and talk to patients! You deal with their immediate medical problems and you jettison everything else and think 'that's my job done, now I'm going home.'

I remember the first thing that struck me when I started being a clinical student was this amazing hierarchy and that senior members, especially surgeons, treated juniors badly. You weren't a person; you were a houseman or a student. There's got to be a radical change in people's attitudes throughout the system... It's very stressful being treated as an 'it', the job is so tough.

If something goes wrong, for instance someone dies, it's very difficult to cope unless you have support... As a student, I often looked at housemen and doctors and how insensitive they were, but now I'm ashamed to say I think I have become part of that process...

I don't think I'm a particularly bad house officer, but only once in the whole ten months has someone told me that I've done something really well, and that was my SHO (Senior House Officer). You never really get positive feedback. I know a lot of junior doctors feel the same. You spend a lot of time feeling you are not getting it right, you should do better, you shouldn't be missing things...

We provide a really awful service...we're so fed up we don't even bother to explain things to patients...I don't understand the more complicated operations which are done, and nobody has bothered to explain them. It's just mindlessly boring...

The study also confirmed the vital yet unrecognized role nurses play in training and supporting junior doctors. As one ward sister put it: 'Consultants are very bad at looking after their own staff. I really resent having to fill the vacuum left by consultants in this area.' Another added, 'In the last week, we have had all the house officers in tears in our office at different times... They are very isolated too. The senior house officers and registrars are often at home at the weekend and may not come out at night.'

Nurses still quietly contribute much to the training of doctors without gaining credit. In September 1998, a staff nurse working on a busy intensive care unit told me, 'It's very stressful keeping an eye on the new doctors. They know nothing about the protocols or how to operate the machines and need a lot of supervision. But if things go wrong, we get the blame.'

Unfortunately for patients, a lot of junior doctors' work is beyond the remit of nurse supervision. For example, house officers still routinely consent patients for surgery and anaesthesia, but a survey of sixty such doctors published in 1996 found that:[3]

- 80 per cent failed to answer correctly simple questions about legal aspects of consent

- 62 per cent had obtained consent from patients on more than five occasions for operations they didn't understand

- 92 per cent had obtained consent from patients whom they thought did not understand the proposed treatments, the possible alternatives and any substantial risk

- None had read the NHS Executive document *A Guide to Consent for Examination and Treatment*

In other words, if you really want to know what's going to happen to you in the operating theatre, don't expect the doctors to tell you automatically.

AFTER HOUSE JOBS
PAEDIATRICS

After my house jobs, in 1988 I secured a place on the Bath GP training scheme. This involved a further two years working in hospital as a senior house officer, and a single year in general practice. When I passed these hurdles, and very few fail, I would be judged fit to work independently as a GP for forty years without any obligation to take further exams or being checked that I've remained up to date, sober and competent.

My first job was as an SHO in paediatrics, working on a special care baby unit. For some as yet unexplained reason, it was considered a good idea for future GPs to know how to ventilate premature babies and insert tiny catheters into tiny umbilical arteries. I've never been brilliant with fine hand movements and I found it very difficult. Fortunately I had a lot of support from my registrars but sometimes they were busy and again it was the nurses who came to the rescue. When I couldn't get a drip or a line in, they would send me away for coffee and when I came back, miraculously it was done. I got the credit because nurses weren't allowed to do such tasks.

I picked up basic skills and there were situations I could manage safely on my own. But the job, by its nature, was unpredictable and no place for a non-specialist. Once I'd been observed doing six successful intubations on newborn babies (putting a tube down into the trachea to help them breath), I was allowed to go to deliveries on my own. Usually all went well but there were two occasions when I couldn't get a tube in. Although senior help was always less than two minutes away, I couldn't help thinking that if someone more experienced had been at the delivery the babies might have done better.

As it was, one died and the other later developed cerebral palsy. Both cases were discussed. The baby who died had serious congenital abnormalities and the baby who developed cerebral palsy had been damaged during the pregnancy. My lack of expertise was not thought though to be a contributory factor in either situation and I was commended for asking for help so quickly. But I felt terrible afterwards. I'm sure one of the main reasons doctors don't blow the whistle on others is because we've all been in situations where our lack of competence may have harmed a patient.

We had a once-a-month staff support group run by a psychologist, where the doctors and nurses working on the special care baby unit were encouraged to talk about how they felt and which deaths had particularly affected them. The nurses sat up at one end in tears and the doctors sat at the other end, embarrassed, staring into their sandwiches and trying not to make eye contact. I decided to keep quiet. Later, I talked it through with another junior paediatrician who was working in a unit with very little support. At night it was just him in the hospital with the consultant at home. He was full of horror stories but when he asked about getting more support he was told, 'You'll just have to fly by the seat of your pants.'

Paediatrics was the toughest job I've ever done, both practically and emotionally. I wasn't cut out for sticking needles into babies and had no preparation for the desperation I felt when a child died of meningitis or cystic fibrosis. I tried hard to be a doctor and not to show frailty or fallibility. I fell back on black humour. I don't think it stopped me caring when I was with patients, but it stopped me going under when I wasn't.

JERSEY

I recovered by moving to Jersey for six months in 1989 to work on a unit which cared for the elderly. At that time, well over 5,000 junior doctors in the UK were working more than eighty-four hours a week. In high-risk specialities (paediatrics, obstetrics and gynaecology, anaesthetics and general surgery) the average was ninety to ninety-five hours.

Part of reason was that we were cheap to employ after hours. In 1989, junior doctors were paid overtime at a third of their basic rate, roughly £1.80 an hour. As a result, the tiredest, most inexperienced doctors were running hospitals and looking after the sickest patients at nights and weekends. A study of house officers in Bristol at that time showed that 85 per cent admitted one or more mistakes and 22 per cent admitted four or more.

The implications are obvious but without systematic audit the scale of the harm done is unclear. In 1987, a Confidential Enquiry into Perioperative Deaths (CEPOD) report of voluntarily reported deaths at or around the time of surgery estimated that about 140 deaths could have been avoided and that the doctor's fatigue was a major factor. In 1990, a review of sixty-four stillbirths, or deaths shortly after birth, that went to litigation found that inadequate foetal heart monitoring, mismanagement of forceps delivery and inadequate supervision by senior staff were contributory factors.

This is only likely to be the tip of the iceberg – CEPOD reporting is only just becoming compulsory and most medical mishaps don't end up in court. In the United States, between 4 and 13 per cent of admissions to hospital are due to medical accidents. Seven per cent of these patients suffer permanent damage and 14 per cent die. In England, where there are about 8 million admissions to hospital a year, even the lower figure would equate to 320,000 medical accidents a year resulting in 40,000 deaths and 20,000 cases of permanent disability.

Despite the hours most junior doctors weren't prepared to complain, but when I discovered that everyone else in the hospital was earning more overtime than the doctors – from the man who picked up the laundry to the woman who rearranged the flowers – I decided the public needed to be told. So I had two thousand 'I Earn More Than My Doctor' badges printed and distributed them around Jersey. They went like hot cakes.

My campaign was on a roll, but the managers were having none of it. They wanted to dig in tight for six months and wait until all the junior doctors rotated round again. So I gave an interview to Channel TV saying that the junior doctors 'would consider taking industrial action' if their pay demands were not met. This was taken to mean that doctors were going on strike, patients panicked and the hospital switchboard was jammed.

A BMA negotiator flew in and after a few terse rounds with the managers, won a 'Jersey waiting allowance' for every junior doctor then and in the future. But the hospital managers could not employ more doctors to bring the hours down, as they had to comply with national guidelines. I was even less happy with the result when I spoke to an elderly patient in the street who hadn't slept for a week because she thought the doctors were going on strike and that she wouldn't get her treatment. But she wanted to give me a donation towards my overtime pay. Slowly I realized whose interests I was supposed to be protecting.

OBSTETRICS

I returned to Bath for six months' worth of obstetrics and gynaecology, and encountered the usual situation of junior doctors dealing with the emergencies. I also met an Australian obstetrician who, although gifted with his hands, was less so with his mouth. Whilst examining the episiotomy cut of a woman who'd just had a baby, he said to her, 'Gee, looks like the mice have been at this.' He then picked up the needle and thread, turned to the husband and said, 'How tight would you like her?'

In Bath, most of the episiotomy repairs were done by the midwives, except the really difficult ones that had torn badly. They were referred to the junior doctors who had never done them before.

PROGRESS IN JUNIOR DOCTOR TRAINING

Until 1996, junior doctors who wanted to become consultants served a series of apprenticeships within so-called consultant 'firms'. Trainees spent ten to fifteen years working long hours and running the health service, rather than receiving structured, supervised training. Patients who were unlucky enough to be treated by often unsupervised doctors at the start of their learning curves undoubtedly got the worst deal. As they rarely complained and the trainees didn't dare do so for fear of ruining a reference, the 'we had to do it and so should you' attitude triumphed for many years.

Recently I spoke to an orthopaedic surgeon who described how, in the 1980s, he and other senior house officers learnt to do hip replacements on their own. He thought he was doing fine until he met his registrar going back to the ward to do his post-operative checks. This involved putting all the hips back in that had fallen out of position after the inept surgery.

The few research studies done so far have found that trainee surgeons produce a much higher rate of complications than the consultants who train them. A study of hip replacements in the *British Journal of Bone Surgery* found that fifteen out of the sixteen patients who required revision arthroplasties (joint replacements), so indicating failure, had been operated on by trainees.[4]

In the past, consultants were kings and could organize their lives according to their individual consciences. Most, like their juniors, put in more hours than they were paid for but a few abused the system and delegated inappropriately complex tasks to trainees while they disappeared to private rooms.

There was a lot of empire building within the hospitals. I know one junior orthopaedic surgeon who tried to do his boss a favour by eliminating the huge waiting list for arthroscopies (internal inspections) of the knee:

I cut it in half, just by eliminating those on the list who'd moved or couldn't be contacted. Half of the remaining patients didn't need to have the procedure at all any more, and for the half that did, I told them to go and 'fall over' outside and I'd see them in casualty and do it as an emergency. I had an anaesthetist who was happy to operate whenever I needed him (we later found out he was a drug addict and was pinching stuff from the trolley, but his anaesthetics were fine). Anyway, I quickly eliminated the waiting list and trotted off to tell my boss the good news. He was not amused. 'Don't you ever, ever, touch my waiting list again. It's my power base within the hospital and my passport to private practice outside.'

Bullying too was common and worse in teaching hospitals. As one consultant told me: 'I've seen consultants punch juniors and once I saw a surgeon deliberately stab a nurse in the hand with his scalpel. Another lifted up his registrar on a ward round and head-butted him in the stomach.'

One advantage of the apprenticeship system was that those doctors who stuck in there long enough to become consultants had usually become very experienced by that time. The irony was that patients did not benefit as much as they might have done from this experience because the new bosses handed over much of the service to their less experienced juniors. The former then lost the skills they'd taken so long to learn and the latter repeated the cycle of learning by trial and error.

In 1996, a new system of structured training was introduced. This was partly to try to improve training and partly to comply with European law, which insists that doctors must obtain their Certificate of Completion of Specialist Training within six years of registration. Consultant firms evolved into clinical teams and juniors were expected to receive training from a wider range of specialists rather than relying heavily on the skills, and reference, of a single consultant.

The training time was further shortened by the reduction in junior doctors' hours. In theory juniors are no longer obliged to do more than fifty-six hours of work a week, although many still do, sometimes willingly. Within this time they are expected to run the service and receive 'quality' training. This quality has remained a myth and, in the words of Junior Doctor Committee chairman Andrew Hobart 'only a relatively small percentage have really good training'. No specialty has got round to defining exactly how the fifty-six hours should be made up.

The ideal would be a consultant-led service, where there are enough experienced specialists to supervise juniors closely and ensure a good service for patients. Unfortunately, we haven't enough consultants so junior doctors are still being left on their own. In 1998, the Confidential Enquiry into Stillbirths and Deaths in Infancy found that most labour wards were run by junior doctors alone. In the consultants' absence 90 per cent of mistakes were made.

In 1997 David Wrede, a senior registrar in obstetrics summed up:

In the current system, the first time you see an obstetric emergency like shoulder dystocia [when the baby's shoulders get stuck] is at night as a green registrar with the consultant at home and unable to assist. If you are lucky, all goes well and you go off duty shaken enough to read everything you can about shoulder dystocia for the next time. If not, the experience haunts you both personally and at the next audit meeting, where you are not usually severely criticized for acting where you had no proven competency.

After five years as a specialist registrar, you may have seen enough cases to feel comfortable managing the condition and then get a consultant post. The irony is that you then do your on-call at home and may never be directly involved in a case again. For the highest quality of care and training in acute specialties, fully trained specialists will have to be resident on-call.

Mr Wrede is adamant about the need for a consultant-led service despite the professional resistance: 'One consultant leader was heard to say "Consultants resident on call? Over my dead body!" Yet if doctors profess to uphold the highest standards of acute care, whose dead bodies are we talking about?'

The NHS is too poor and understaffed to provide a widespread, quality service for all, and there are many published studies showing that junior doctors are not getting the training they need, despite a plethora of guidelines from important bodies. In 1993 the Royal College of Surgeons stated that 'All doctors involved in the initial resuscitation and management of patients with major illnesses should possess a current Advanced Trauma Life Support Provider Certificate. But a study of SHOs working in the 13 major accident and emergency departments in the South-west region found that, in 1994, only 16 per cent did and, in 1995, only 11 per cent did.

A study by Cardiff Royal Infirmary involved a random telephone survey of 113 doctors in cardiac arrest teams from sixty-two teaching and district general hospitals in England and Wales. Only thirty-two knew the full sequence of managing ventricular fibrillation (the commonest cause of cardiac arrest) and thirty-two didn't even know the initial actions to take.[5]

These poor results occurred despite previous warnings that that the resuscitation skills of house officers and candidates for membership of the Royal College of Physicians were very poor.[6] In the latter study, a staggering twenty-nine out of thirty candidates 'neglected fundamental rules for the management of cardiac arrest.' They lacked knowledge of basic life support skills and Resuscitation Council Guidelines for arrest management, drug treatment and defibrillation.

This is all the more unsettling because there is clear evidence that the survival of patients suffering cardiac arrest is directly linked to the attending doctor's skills and knowledge of the correct treatment, the availability of working resuscitation equipment and coordination with other team members.[7]

Training in paediatric resuscitation is also poor.[8] When questionnaires were sent to the on-call paediatric senior house officer covering the labour ward at 100 British hospitals it was found that none of the respondents had been on an advanced paediatric or advanced trauma life support course. Generally, they were expected 'to learn on the job.' Forty respondents thought their training was inadequate or 'very basic', twenty-one did not feel confident about intubation, ten had had to summon help urgently during resuscitation owing to their inability to maintain an airway and six had been the only doctor immediately available during resuscitation.

An investigation of deaths of babies under one month old found that in more than half the cases different care 'would reasonably have been expected to have made a difference' and in a further 25 per cent of cases it 'might have made a difference.'[9]

The report recommended improved supervision of junior staff and called for nationally approved assessment and accreditation of the relevant staff.

A year later, the fifth annual Confidential Enquiry into Stillbirths and Deaths confirmed that some babies die due to 'poor clinical management'. Many of the babies who died had been ill enough to warrant medical attention in the twenty-four hours before they died, but appropriate action was not taken. The single most common reason why babies died outside hospital was the GPs' failure to recognize the severity of the illness. Three deaths also occurred after babies had been seen and discharged by a junior doctor without a senior opinion. The well-documented and widespread occurrence of preventable deaths in babies lends some weight to the claims of the Bristol heart surgeons that they have been made scapegoats for a much wider problem.

Adults also receive patchy quality care. A study in the *BMJ* in 1998 found that half of the patients admitted to hospital in 1992–93 in an emergency received poor care which doubles their risk of dying. Major factors included delays in treatment, poor management of breathing and circulation problems and inadequate monitoring of the patients' condition. Junior doctors in particular failed to appreciate urgency, lacked supervision, failed to seek advice, had poor knowledge and didn't appreciate 'the pre-requisites of life'.[10]

Another recurrent theme is that when new equipment arrives, doctors often start using it without much structured training. A study of eighty-five surgical trainees in the west of Scotland found that although all had assisted and most had performed laparoscopic surgery, only eighteen had attended a structured training course.[11]

Another BMJ study compared laparoscopic and traditional 'open' inguinal hernia repair. The new technology had a complication rate of 12 per cent at an average cost of £850, while the traditional method had a complication rate of 2 per cent and an average cost of £268. Both groups returned to normal activity at the same time.[12] Defenders of the laparoscopic method pointed out that the problem was the technique or poor training of the surgeons rather than the method itself.

In June 1996, *The Doctors Tale Continued*, published by the Audit Commission, found that:

- A quarter of weekend and night operations, usually emergencies, are carried out by unsupervised junior doctors

- Only a quarter of consultants always supervised their SHOs

- One in five house officers and one in ten SHOs perform at least one task a week (including operations) they feel is beyond their competence

- Only 50 per cent of consultants attend all outpatient clinics

- 20 per cent of consultants freely admitted that they did not discuss any patients with their junior doctors

Another study published in the *BMJ* found that senior house officers were often left alone to do their first salivary gland excisions, hernia repairs and stomach, spleen and gall bladder removals, with senior 'support' not present in the hospital, while surgical registrars were carrying out complex and life threatening first-time surgery of the liver, gall bladder and pancreas, often in emergency situations. Emergency bowel resections, leaking aortic aneurysms and a kidney transplant were also being done for the first time unsupervised.

There will always be situations when surgeons have to muddle through for lack of support. In some cases, however, support should have been available and was not, either because consultants were at home in bed or at a private hospital or in a neighbouring theatre desperately trying to get the waiting lists down. As for the consultants, five out of the seventeen general surgical consultants had performed a procedure not seen during training and seven had performed procedures that they had only assisted at in training.

Clearly every consultant will not have mastered every procedure in their specialty before they qualify, but they may be able to transfer their skills to new procedures and do them competently. Changes in medical training and the reduction in junior doctors' hours mean that juniors become consultants more quickly. So the risk of excessive 'first-time' surgery for young consultants will increase. In the survey, thirty-eight head and neck procedures had been performed by surgeons who had never previously seen them.

Interestingly, many of the studies cited here were published several years after the research took place, giving rise to the suspicion that, despite the time needed to collate the research, delaying tactics are being used to prevent such unsettling information getting into the public domain. The time lapse also allows eminent surgeons to say that training has improved since the time of the study.

It is much easier to claim things are improving if there is no public audit of your work. It is very rare in surgery, and indeed medicine as a whole, for results to be collected and processed in a meaningful form that allows comparisons between doctors or hospitals. Many surgeons do not want to know. Any admission that a surgeon is going off the boil or should no longer be attempting certain more difficult procedures can have knock-on effects for private work, and many consultants still have large debts into their mid fifties. Given that there is no obligation to prove either that an operation is effective or that you are competent to do it, it is far easier to carry on in blissful ignorance.

Most doctors are competent, but at present we have no means of proving it and so it is hard to protect patients from the few doctors who are not fit to practice or, more commonly, from those who are competent but occasionally over-stretch themselves. The lack of public safeguards and accountability is highlighted by the ease with which bogus doctors slot into the NHS and 'practise' undetected for years.

BOGUS DOCTORS, AND WHAT THEY MEAN

The scale of this problem is not great, but the fact that there are more than a hundred documented cases is alarming.[13] We doctors are selected as the top 0.1 per cent of the academic population, and we like to think the successful practice of medicine is the summit of knowledge, skill and intellect, requiring prolonged, arduous training and enormous moral integrity. So how can anyone possibly fake it?

With relative ease, is the answer. On *Trust Me (I'm a Doctor)* we interviewed a bogus doctor called John, who left school without exams and after a brief stint as a hospital orderly began a long a successful bogus career as an NHS doctor.[14] He started as a locum orthopaedic house officer without giving any references (the hospital was desperately understaffed). John didn't look out of place and subsequently secured a job as a senior house officer in orthopaedics on the strength of a verbal reference from his consultant. He assisted with operations and even did a few himself.

He then decided to have a stint at anaesthetics at another hospital. Although he asked for help more often than seemed necessary, this was viewed as a good thing. He continued in anaesthetics at yet another hospital (by this time he had a string of good references) and his work was judged satisfactory. He became a registrar at one of his previous hospitals and even passed his fellowship exams in anaesthetics.

Finally he progressed to senior registrar and then locum consultant. No one complained. As Dr Mike Norman, a real consultant anaesthetist who worked with John put it: 'Everybody was very pleased with his work... I was very, very surprised that he wasn't a doctor, because he conducted himself as if he was. He had access to all kinds of patients, babies and children. He was particularly good with children... I can never remember anything going wrong or any disasters at all. And I'm sure I would have heard if people had said, "Oh, we don't want John to give anaesthetics".'

John, too, was confident about his ability: 'I know all doctors will hate me for saying this, but it's not a difficult profession to practise really. There are only a certain number of things that can go wrong with you, a bit like a car...' In casualty he dealt with 'lacerations, cardiac arrests, broken bones, road traffic accidents and a lot of petty stuff, rashes and things. It just comes through the door and you deal with it.'

But it was in anaesthetics where he shone. 'By the time I was a registrar I was getting real doctors out of trouble. They had fellowships and memberships and diplomas but when it actually came to hands on they were abysmal, some of them dreadful.' John was eventually offered a permanent consultant post but never took it up. He was rumbled not for his doctoring, but for taking part in a bogus insurance scam. If he hadn't become greedy he might possibly have been President of the Royal College of Anaesthetists by now.

Lessons to be learnt from cases like John's are that:

- Both patients and NHS staff are alarmingly trusting of anyone in a white coat.

- Most bogus hospital doctors start in junior posts and remain undetected even if they're terrible. The reason is that medical education and training are so poor that many consultants expect their most junior staff to be incompetent. House officers are supposed to be clumsy, ignorant and dangerous despite five years at medical school.

- The medical profession and the whole NHS system colludes in concealing errors so protecting both its real and bogus staff.

- Hospitals with staff shortages can be hoodwinked into taking on impostors through desperation. In the past, bogus doctors got away with no references and forged certificates, even poor quality photocopies. Today photocopies are not supposed to be accepted and hospitals are advised to check with the GMC.

- Given the shortage of doctors, does it matter if a bogus doctor carries on practising if a review of his work shows him – most bogus doctors are men – to be as good as if not better than real doctors?

- If bogus doctors are as good as John, it's difficult for patients to spot them. Even if they aren't, it's still very rare for patients to challenge them. The UK record for impersonating a doctor is held by Mohammed Saed, who was a bogus GP in Bradford for thirty years before he was caught. He prescribed shampoo for conjunctivitis, creosote for a sore throat and cough linctus to be rubbed into the scalp. His patients did not complain, and although a pharmacist tried to raise the alarm, he was passed fit to practise by a peer review from two medical colleagues. He was eventually shopped by a relative.

MORE STRESS AND ALCOHOL

In 1987, a *BMJ* study found that 28 per cent of house officers registered clinical depression, with those in teaching hospitals being significantly more stressed. The toughest aspects of their jobs were 'overwork, talking to distressed relatives, effects on personal life, serious treatment failures and relations with consultants.'[15]

Since then, there have been numerous studies highlighting the stress among junior doctors. In 1991, a study of doctors who qualified in 1986 found that 58 per cent of men and 76 per cent of women regretted entering medicine.[16]

A study by doctors at the Tavistock Clinic found that if young doctors ever had the capacity for reflection and introspection, many of them lose it. When asked to relate an episode about five significant people in their life, many found the task virtually impossible. They stalled, laughed to disguise embarrassment and when they did articulate any experiences, trivialized them. They had lost the capacity to think, reflect, feel and articulate with any depth.[17]

So what happens to doctors further down the life cycle? Physically, we are healthier than average, but mentally we're often shot to pieces. We're especially prone to mental illness such as depression, drug addiction and alcoholism. 'Psychologically related deaths', including suicide, 'accidental' poisoning and cirrhosis are also higher than average and higher than other professions except dentists.[18]

Drinking and drug abuse are clearly coping mechanisms picked up in medical school, but it is impossible to predict which of the many heavy student drinkers will go on to develop a problem. We covered this topic in *Trust Me (I'm a Doctor)*[19] after the BMA estimated that up to 13,000 practising UK doctors are addicted to drugs or alcohol. Despite the existence of numerous support agencies to help doctors, the vast majority never come to their attention. Most addicted doctors hide behind their status and conceal their habits. Colleagues, if they suspect a problem, often don't raise the alarm. Action is only taken if a clinical disaster happens or, more usually, if the doctor is done for drunk driving.

Even then, action taken may not sort out the problem. Dr Ian Joiner is a recovering alcoholic who, for thirty-five years, was drinking between three and four bottles of gin a week. He was convicted of drink-driving four times and placed under psychiatric supervision for seven years. His experience of the ineffectiveness of this prompted him to set up his own Addicted Physicians Programme in July 1995. He told me of 'a heart surgeon who was drinking half a bottle of vodka a day so that he could steady his hands before he could perform an operation. He was unable to take my advice, saw a psychiatrist locally and he's still out there, still practising.'

Just as nobody's sure who the good, bad and bogus doctors are, we also have no way of knowing what damage the 13,000 addicted doctors do to patients. If each make 2,000 clinical decisions a year, at a conservative estimate, that is 26 million decisions affecting patient care made by doctors who can't function without alcohol or other drugs.

In 1998, I spoke to a surgeon about the stresses of working with an alcoholic colleague:

> We knew he had a problem and for a while we covered up for him until the workload got too much. Then we insisted he get help through the 'three wise men' system [which requires hospital medical staff committees to set up a panel of three doctors to consider cases in which a doctor's illness or disability may be a danger to patients]. He was allowed to carry on operating with psychiatric support and supervision of his work.
>
> Some months later, I discovered that I was the one who was supposed to be supervising the work but no one had told me. In any case, I was too busy doing his work for him and undoing his mistakes to monitor him. We kept trying to get him to stop operating because he was a risk to patients but it took ten years, from start to finish, before he agreed to stop and then only because he'd started to have fits.

The GMC has highlighted the duty of doctors to own up to their own problems and blow the whistle on problem colleagues, but it remains to be seen if this will happen. Admitting to alcoholism is a huge stigma in medicine and sufferers fear that seeking treatment is a passport to career ruin. Ironically, there is evidence from America that doctors do extremely well in expert rehab programmes (rather than the current ad hoc supervision in the NHS) and can safely return to work.

There is a sense too that doctors are in part their own worst enemies. We take in obsessive, compulsive over-achievers at a young age and teach them that ignorance and expressions of emotion are signs of weakness. They develop a misplaced, arrogant certainty about medicine, unrealistic expectations of their future and tunnel vision towards an impossible goal. More importantly, many have an inability to tolerate uncertainty. We develop what's known as 'the mask of relaxed brilliance' to help us appear competent when we haven't got a clue, just as we learn to appear sober with a distillery coursing through our veins. Workaholism is seen as an attribute, rather than an illness, and if we're lucky enough to survive and make it to the top, we're only too keen to inflict more of the same on our junior staff. As one consultant confided in me: 'Once you've sacrificed your marriage and your liver to become a consultant, you don't want the buggers underneath you to find an easier route'.

POSTGRADUATE MEDICAL HUMOUR

As a house officer at Frenchay Hospital in Bristol in 1987, I asked three first-year student nurses to write a song for the Christmas Show. They were working on a care of the elderly ward and decided to rewrite the lyrics of 'Merry Christmas Ev'rybody' by Slade. The chorus went:

So here it is Geriatrics
Ev'rybody's had a stroke
Let's get the turkey out
And see how many choke

Most doctors believe that patients should be protected from this sort of humour, that it should stay in the sluice room or behind the closed doors of medical school. But I believe that if you want to understand doctors and nurses, the type of people we are and what our work does to us, you need to understand our humour. Whenever I've tried to raise this subject, I've been shot down for exaggeration. They're only jokes after all.

But do these attitudes dictate behaviour? I've heard elderly patients referred to as crud, crap, crumble, bed-blockers, TF BUNDY (Totally Fucked But Unfortunately Not Dead Yet) and JP FROG (Just Plain Fucking Run Outta Gas). Women have been referred to as GROLIES (Guardian Readers of Limited Intelligence in Ethnic Skirts) and a clinic a friend worked in for women with hormone disorders was nicknamed the FHWC (Fat Hairy Woman Clinic).

In casualty, some patients are PAFO (Pissed And Fell Over) and there are OAPs (Over-Anxious Parents) and SIGs (Stroppy, Ignorant Gits). Some abbreviations have pejorative regional overlay. If you work in Winchester, cerebrally challenged patients are NFA (Normal for Andover), in Taunton they're NFB (Normal for Bridgwater) and in Norwich they're NFN (Normal for Norfolk). None of these abbreviations appear in the notes, although prior to the Freedom of Information Act, which allows patients to read parts of their post-1990 notes, written insults weren't that uncommon. For example, a Bristol gynaecologist wrote to a GP about a very large woman on whom he had tried and failed to perform a D&C: 'I regret that I'm unable to perform this procedure without the aid of a miner's lamp and a canary.'

A lot of the humour revolves around men abusing women. I trained with a doctor who wanted to be an obstetrician because he enjoyed 'womb wiggling'. One of my GP partners was taught by an obstetrician who, after every examination, would tweak the woman's pubic hair before leaving the room. And a consultant obstetrician in London used to counter women who claimed their pregnancy was an accident with: 'An accident, was it? So you're telling me, you were walking down the high street, you tripped on a loose paving slab and fell onto an erect penis?'

Whilst I applaud the Royal College of Obstetricians and Gynaecologists for their 1997 guidelines on how their members should behave during intimate examinations, when I recently asked a room full of gynaecologists if any could name them only one could, and he helped write them. After my talk a consultant came across to tell me about a colleague who did a lot of fertility treatment. 'When he wasn't getting results, he used to slip a bit of his own sperm into the samples. You can use that if you like. He's dead now.'

One actor I know was admitted to hospital with abdominal pain and had a gratuitous rectal examination done by a surgeon 'for a laugh'. I discovered this when I met his colleague who said, 'All the team got together in the mess to see who had the biggest fingers. He won by a mile and did it very thoroughly.'

I'm sure this sort of abuse is very rare, but the point is that when rare but serious abuses happen in medicine, from unnecessary examinations to incompetent surgery, the culture has been cover up and, in some cases, celebrate. Recently I met a cardiologist who told me of a medical registrar he worked with who used to perform unnecessary sigmoidoscopies (rectal examinations with a steel tube) on elderly patients who were blocking beds. He'd point the sigmoidoscope like a gun and say, 'Right, who's going to ride the silver rocket today?' It was apparently very effective in getting people moving. His colleagues thought this highly amusing.

As a student, I queued to do internal examinations on unconscious women without their consent. This particular practice is now frowned upon, but is it any better when you know what's going on? A GP I know described lining up with seven other students to examine an elderly man's prostate gland. To make it kinder to the patient's sphincter, one student's finger had to stay in while the next student's finger slid over it before the first withdrew. And this while the consultant was shouting '*en glissade, en glissade*'.

Are GPs any kinder? We might rate highly in household surveys but Tony Copperfield, a pseudonymous GP created by several real ones, paints a pretty bleak picture of family practice in a weekly column for *Doctor* magazine.[20] For instance, for difficult patients, he suggests GPs should 'blast that abusive moron away with a sawn-off 12-bore shotgun'. Dr C is 'sick of being nice…I want to be able to shout at stupid patients, tell my heartsinks what I really feel about them, insult middle class mothers who believe little Gemma has a food allergy… I have decided to make the great sacrifice of being horrible to all of my patients all of the time.' For him '…patients are ungrateful, manipulative, rude scumbags' to whom he would like to 'hand out a practice advice leaflet saying "sod off"'.

When doctors get together we love recounting real live horror stories, like the one about the doctor who gave his patient too much diamorphine and she stopped breathing. He asked the nurse for the antidote, Naloxone, and she misheard him and handed him Lanoxin, a heart drug. Without realizing the error, he administered ampoule after ampoule of the drug, not understanding why it wasn't working. The patient died and the cock up was covered up.

In 1994, ex-junior doctor Ged Mercurio brought this brutal, self-protective image of medicine to television for the first time in BBC 2's *Cardiac Arrest.* An NHS hospital was depicted as a war zone, with the staff bullying each other, humiliating patients and taking the path of least resistance in order to survive. The only way to cope was not to care.

For the first time in a British TV programme, nurses were portrayed as a bunch of clock-watching, bolshy witches and the rougher side of doctors was shown. A junior doctor performed a deliberately harsh catheterization and filled the balloon (the thing that holds the catheter in) with tea. Another made easily overheard remarks about a man with lung cancer ('he's got so much asbestos in him it'll take a year to cremate him'). A bullied female doctor with an alcohol problem committed suicide. All very bleak and unsettling.

On the whole, doctors loved it and one survey of juniors judged it to be an accurate portrayal of their working conditions.[21] But a lot of patients didn't want to believe it. On the eve of your prostate operation, do you want to see poorly trained, knackered, unsupervised junior doctors stalking the wards, maiming patients through misadventure and making inappropriate jokes about death? The series started with 10 million viewers and went steadily downhill, despite desperate attempts to inject more empathy in subsequent series. As one critic put it, 'If this really is the NHS, then it isn't worth saving.'

My own view is that, despite their lapses into black humour, most doctors do care. I would be quite happy to trust a surgeon who sometimes laughs at his patients provided he's doesn't so all the time and, most important of all, that he's technically (if not emotionally) competent.

However, where medical humour becomes sinister is where it acts as a mask or manifestation of incompetence. Not only was Kent gynaecologist Rodney Ledward nicknamed The Butcher, but he billed himself as 'the fastest gynaecologist in the South East' after completing seven hysterectomies between 8a.m. and noon. He is also alleged to have turned up for operations and walked onto wards wearing hunting gear and jodhpurs.

In striking him off in September 1998, the GMC found that he ignored 'basic medical procedures' and gave treatment that was 'inappropriate' or had 'no scientific basis'. His errors were so gross that some patients almost bled to death and had to be patched up by colleagues. Many of the staff at William Harvey Hospital in Kent and the private hospitals he worked at must have known about his incompetence before he was finally suspended. Why did they not step in to protect patients? Were they frightened of him? Were they friends with him? Or did they share his cavalier sense of humour?

I have only once worked with a colleague whose competence was such that I wouldn't let him near my family. He was a registrar in gynaecology and was even clumsier than I am with my hands. But whereas I asked for help for anything that I knew was beyond my capability, he didn't. On one occasion, he made such a mess of a forceps delivery that the woman had to go to theatre to be sutured. The senior registrar was fuming: 'What the hell have you done? It looks like a grenade's gone off in here.'

The registrar was eventually counselled out of a career as a surgeon, but others escape censure for their 'mistakes'. In *The Citadel Lancet* editor Richard Horton told the President of the Royal College of Surgeons that 'a senior member of your own college' had cut a patient's ureter in half just to teach a junior how to stitch it back together again.[22] The President, Sir Rodney Sweetnam, replied: 'I frankly don't believe it. I'm sorry...I cannot accept that.'

I can. In 1997 I spoke to a student who had witnessed two junior surgeons racing each other in adjacent theatres to perform an axillary clearance operation to remove lymph glands under the arm in women with breast cancer. One was technically proficient and achieved a good result. The other wasn't; he punctured a blood vessel and the woman needed a blood transfusion and a return to theatre. I asked the student to name the hospital and the surgeons so the matter could be investigated but he was too frightened.

He was only working briefly on a surgical attachment, had no way of proving what had happened other than his own testimony and was just glad to get out of there. But what if you are employed in a unit where the mortality rates seems inexplicably high every year? And what if babies are dying? How do you cope with that? Do you risk your career and blow the whistle? Or do you just keep silent?

3 | PUBLISH AND BE PRAISED

'Before the Department of Health bestows its mark of excellence on the United Bristol Healthcare Trust, it may wish to ponder the perilous state of its paediatric cardiac surgery. In 1988, the mortality was so high the unit was dubbed 'The Killing Fields'. Despite a long crisis of morale among intensive care staff, the surgeons persistently refuse to publish their mortality rates in a manner comparable to other units...'

Private Eye, *May 8, 1992*

'Investigations of the events at the Bristol Royal Infirmary were started by the GMC itself in April 1996 following an article in *The Times* by Lord Rees-Mogg... The Professional Conduct Committee found two surgeons had continued to perform certain operations despite growing concerns about poor mortality figures. They did not adequately establish the causes of those results. One of them misled parents about likely outcomes. And the then chief executive failed to take action when colleagues voiced anxieties...'

Summer 1998 edition of *General Medical Council News*, reporting on an investigation into heart operations on fifty-three children and babies at the Bristol Royal Infirmary between 1988 and 1995. Twenty-nine died and four were left brain damaged.

'The work of these two surgeons has been scrutinized more than any other doctor's in the history of the GMC. Many of the charges against them were dropped and those that stuck relate to only 4 per cent of the operations they carried out on children. Surely if you painstakingly examine the work of any surgeon, any doctor even, you can find a small area where the results are disappointing. By that measure every doctor in the UK is incompetent.'

A consultant reviewing the GMC verdict

'Roger Henderson, QC for the GMC, said that Mr Wisheart should have realized by 1993 that the mortality of up to 54 per cent associated with the operations he carried out to correct atrioventricular septal defects – compared with the national average of 13.9 per cent – was "comparatively disastrous."'

British Medical Journal, *18 October 1997 pp 967*

'What went on at Bristol was not seen by my generation as so terrible a thing while it was happening. It was identified by a younger generation as an incorrect way of practising.'

*Professor Arnold Maran, president of the Royal College of Surgeons of Edinburgh (*Hospital Doctor, *29 October 1998)*

'Parents used to say, "See you later" to their children and I used to stand there thinking, "No, you won't".'

*Whistle-blowing nurse Helen Stratton (*Health Service Journal, *4 June, 1998)*

'The results for the [Bristol] unit in 1997–8 are excellent as well as comprehensive and show that we are functioning as a cardiac surgical unit of the highest quality. There is no difference between the performance of any of the current surgical teams. The full audit documents for both adult and paediatric cardiac surgery... will be made publicly available shortly.'

'Cardiac services in Bristol are now of high quality' (*BMJ*, 27 June 1998 p1986)

"

Although I'd heard rumours about the poor performance of an adult heart surgeon (nicknamed 'Killer') in Bristol when I was a house officer in Bath, there were no such rumours about paediatric heart surgery. When I spoke to one of my former consultants in November 1998, he said they had never heard anything bad about the Bristol unit until 1995, when the mainstream media finally caught up with *Private Eye*.

However, he did say that when he worked at the Hammersmith Hospital in London in 1985, he noticed an abnormal referral pattern coming out of South Wales. Babies with more complex heart defects requiring surgery appeared to be bypassing the Bristol area. This was corroborated by an anaesthetist who worked on the paediatric cardiac surgery unit at Guy's Hospital in the late 1980s. He noticed that his unit, and the unit at the Royal Brompton Hospital, were receiving many difficult referrals from Cardiff and the South West. When he asked the referring doctors why they did not send them to the nearby unit in Bristol, he was told, 'Difficult cases die in Bristol. So we only send them the easy ones.'

This pattern of doctors far away from Bristol realizing there was something wrong with the paediatric heart surgery unit but those closer to home not having a clue is one of the most perplexing things about this tragedy. A consultant paediatric gastroenterologist who works at Bristol Children's Hospital told me: 'We honestly had no suspicion at all that anything bad was happening. I suppose it was because, although we may have been working in the same building, specialities often don't mix at all. I would know if someone was mucking up the endoscopes but I wouldn't necessarily know about heart surgery.'

I came to be involved in exposing the Bristol tragedy in an unconventional way – via stand-up comedy. In January 1990 I teamed up with Tony Gardner, a fellow junior doctor, to form 'Struck Off and Die'. We had two naïve beliefs – that we could make a difference to the working conditions of junior doctors through comedy, and that the best way to demystify medicine was to get people to understand medical humour: it's black, it's cruel but it's not our fault – you should see the system we have to work in. And for those who didn't like it and preferred to think of doctors as gods and nurses as super-human caring machines, we used John Cleese's defence of *Life of Brian*: 'Some people deserve to be offended.'

We went up to the Edinburgh Fringe and performed for three weeks in a sweaty Masonic Lodge on the Royal Mile. We got lots of reviews, good and bad. Fortunately the good ones came before the bad, so we sold out every night, got work on BSkyB and a promise of a Radio 4 series. We were hooked. Subsequently, we did two Radio 4 series, won a few awards, found an agent and continued to sell out. We also made a lot of junior doctors laugh in recognition ('the reason we draw the curtains around a patient's bed when he dies, is so the doctor can raid the fruit bowl without anybody noticing').

In between the smut, we wrote satirical sketches about the sexism, racism, and classism in medicine, the crap surgeons and dangerous juniors, the secrecy, the Stalinist macho managers, the sinister politicians who kill far more people than doctors and the 'un-science' of what we do. But they were only ever sketches. As one consultant anaesthetist warned me, 'Your job is to entertain. Don't ever start taking it seriously.'

By 1991, Tony and I had become minor medical celebrities and, after picketing the Conservative Party conference in support of junior doctors in Blackpool, we were invited to write a column for *Hospital Doctor* called 'Joblot'. The idea was to provide a confidential whistle-blowing forum for junior doctors who were too frightened to speak out.

The complaints were depressingly repetitive. A junior psychiatrist in London was on duty for 196 hours in twelve days (including 136 hours on call), but was refused a half day off by his consultant and chief executive. Surgical house officers in Newcastle were doing 150 hours on duty when colleagues were on holiday, SHOs at the Royal Alexandra Hospital for Sick Children were doing 'a ludicrously dangerous on-call week' and so on.

The implication was obvious: patients suffer and die for lack of well-trained doctors – as well as a lack of nurses and resources – but no one has ever wanted to be too explicit for fear of being branded a scare-mongerer. We could do it in comic sketches but, like *Cardiac Arrest*, people didn't want to know the reality. Also, it is extremely difficult to prove that patients die because of patchy quality care because, until the Bristol tragedy, there had been no obligation, and little inclination, to audit the work.

This was partly because good, fair audit is expensive and time consuming, and not many people had the resources or stamina to do it. It also requires a major cultural shift away from the view that 'we're all bloody good chaps and our best is good enough, so why bother with audit?' to that of 'the doctor's best needs to be above an agreed standard of minimal competence.' Given the patchy standard of training, poor working conditions and lack of resources in the NHS, audit was, and is, bound to uncover unpalatable truths about the quality of the service that are hard to address.

Ironically given what happened in Bristol, heart surgery was one of the first disciplines to embrace the idea of collecting activity and mortality figures. Since 1977, a UK register has collected basic information about the 35,000 or so operations that are carried out in NHS heart surgery units. This is clearly a good thing, since millions of pounds of public money go into the specialty and the results can be catastrophic if not done well.

However, submission of the data was voluntary, not every death was tracked down and the information was kept anonymous to encourage units to hand it over. The theory was that the staff in each surgical unit could gain access to their own information, compare it to national data, and take appropriate action if performance was not up to the mark.

Individual doctors who submitted data could not be identified by others, and might not even be able to spot themselves, given that the data related to surgical units, rather than to individuals. This rightly recognized that cardiac surgery is complex, operations are a team effort and the outcome depends on the combined skills of the cardiologist, anaesthetist, surgeon and nursing staff as well as their equipment and facilities. However, a unit's figures can easily mask a single poor performer.

Audit is only any use if it's acted on. After the GMC verdict, Tom Treasure, a cardiac surgeon at St George's Hospital, London, cited the 'unheard warnings' about Bristol from a 1989 audit led by Professor David Hamilton and the UK register for paediatric cardiac surgery.[1] Why was no action taken?

Figures alone are not enough. One of the crucial issues in allowing fair comparison between individual surgeons and units is to allow for something called 'case-mix'. If you take on the hardest operations on the sickest patients, your results are likely to be worse than those who take on easier operations. This can be adjusted for by a statistical process called risk stratification, which depends for its success on someone compiling an accurate risk profile of the patient and the surgery they are due to undergo.

Releasing 'unstratified' figures about a unit's performance, without adjusting for case-mix, is clearly not ideal. In the United States, when the Freedom of Information Act came in and forced these raw results into the public domain, it caused considerable panic. Some units were unfairly branded as poor for taking on the hardest cases, and some were praised when in fact they had cherry picked the easy ones. Without a fair means of comparison, surgeons might just refuse to operate on the sickest patients.

Risk stratification allows a fair comparison and highlights a surgical unit performing poorly but wrongly blaming the results on the severity of the patients' condition.

In the UK, the Society of Cardiothoracic Surgeons began risk-stratified audit in 1993, but again – and this I find extraordinary given that the problems in Bristol were widely known within the specialty by that time – it was not compulsory and individual surgeons were not identified. This, according to an editorial in the *BMJ* 'would have been an insurmountable stumbling block to its launch.'[2] In 1998, data was accepted from only just over half of all the British units. So bad units could again lie undiscovered. This database was also set up for adults only; only since 1998 has a paediatric surgical database been developed.

Most specialties are way behind cardiothoracic surgery in data collection and audit, so we haven't a clue what cock-ups may have happened in the past and we still can't be sure what's happening in many units. Poor performers have generally only been spotted if they have had such bad results across the board that they are obviously a danger to patients. Even then, it can take many years before they are forced to stop, partly because of the reluctance of doctors to shop their colleagues and partly because no one has defined standards of minimal competence, let alone collected solid evidence to distinguish acceptable from unacceptable.

The flip side of this is that doctors who have been suspended because of a vendetta or some other professional jealousy often have a great deal of difficulty proving their competence. In the majority of cases of suspension, the case is never proven but suspension can drag on for years, destroying the doctors' lives and costing a fortune to the NHS in wages.

An oncologist I spoke to was suspended for giving a patient the wrong dose of chemotherapy. It was his first offence, and an investigation found that the fifteen minutes per patient he was allowed to calculate the right dose was grossly inadequate. He remained suspended, but because the hospital couldn't find a locum to replace him, his colleagues had to cover his workload. So patients only got twelve minutes each plus an increased risk of further mistakes.

In 1988, the Department of Health declared 'there are no plans to require regular self-assessment by clinicians'. Ten years, and a huge tragedy later, the government finally announced a compulsory systematic audit as part of the system of clinical governance. It remains to be seen whether it will be given the resources to do the job effectively and, crucially, how much will be publicized. And in my view, as soon as good, risk-stratified audit has been prepared and statistically verified it should be published.

Secrecy, of course, is not the exclusive domain of the medical profession. It is just as bad in Government and the civil service. As the former Prime Minister Edward Heath pointed out, Britain is the most secretive of all the Western democracies and the habit of telling its citizens as little as possible is ingrained in the ruling classes.

It remains to be seen whether the Labour government delivers its promise of a Freedom of Information Act. It was absent from the Queen's Speech to mark the opening of Parliament on 24 November 1998 and, if it does appear, it is likely to be watered down.

In 1988, the Department of Health carried out an audit of paediatric heart surgery in the UK and found that the Bristol unit was doing fewer than average open-heart operations on children and that the mortality rate was the highest of all the nine specialist units. The humane response would have been to suspend operations and investigate further, or at the very least make the information available to parents to allow them to make informed choices. Instead the DoH kept the audit unpublished and advised the unit to carry out more of the operations.

In-house audit was also carried out each month by the Bristol team – surgeons, cardiologists, radiologists, anaesthetists and pathologists. However, the whistle-blowing anaesthetist Steve Bolsin complained that figures were not prepared in a way that allowed valid comparison with other units and, for the two years with the highest mortality, they were not presented to the board or the purchasers. This perhaps explains why some doctors working in close proximity to the unit never got to hear about the problems.

'Wisheart was in charge of audit at the hospital,' said Bolsin. 'If you control all the avenues of power you can dictate what information is circulated.'[3] His complaints were dismissed by the hospital management and, as an acknowledged expert in audit techniques, he decided to conduct his own audit without the cooperation of those he was auditing.

I was alerted to the problems in February 1992. Three months previously I'd met Ian Hislop, the editor of *Private Eye*, at a BBC Radio Light Entertainment Christmas Party and asked him if he would like a medical correspondent. My joint column in *Hospital Doctor* had been a success but it was for doctors only. I was convinced the public should be told what was going on. I wanted to keep the whistle-blowing forum for NHS workers and add in the experiences of *Eye* readers.

Hislop said I'd have to use a pseudonym, and for professional and legal reasons, I accepted this condition. I was still a junior doctor with no experience of journalism and if I screwed up the *Eye* would survive but my medical career would be over. The use of a pseudonym also allowed other journalists to contribute to the column. The downside, as I later discovered, was that although *Private Eye* is the closest thing to a free press we have in this country, the anonymity of authorship as much as the satire allows it to be dismissed.

In February 1992, I started work as a casualty officer in Taunton, while Tony Gardner took up a similar post at the Bristol Royal Infirmary. We'd both done our house jobs in Bristol and, as a result, had lots of contacts there. Perhaps not surprisingly, Bristol hospitals received an unfair amount of emphasis in *Private Eye*.

To understand what went on with child heart surgery at the Bristol Royal Infirmary (part of the then newly formed United Bristol Healthcare Trust), it is worth remembering that it is a teaching hospital. So, alongside all the cutting-edge medicine are also secrecy, odd personalities, workaholism, arrogance, professional jealousy, empire building, lack of insight and institutional loyalty. The loyalty in Bristol is compounded by the fact that many of the consultants had known each other 'man and boy' and were close friends.

Equally important is to place the events in their political context. In 1983 Sir Roy Griffiths, Sainsbury's managing director, led an inquiry into management in the NHS. His report stated: 'If Florence Nightingale were carrying her lamp through the corridors of the NHS she would almost certainly be searching for the people in charge.' This clearly irked Margaret Thatcher, the then Prime Minister, who instituted the health reforms which led to the formation of hospital into so-called 'Trusts' (new corporate image, new costumes, new note-paper, new mission statement).

The result of the reforms was that hospitals had to compete with each other for money from 'purchasers', namely Health Authorities and fund-holding GPs. They had to balance the books or heads would roll. So no one wanted to look too hard for poor quality, which might put off the purchasers, and if some fool brought it to your attention, you buried it for as long as possible.

In this context many hospitals operated in a climate of fear. Job contracts contained gagging clauses. Articles appeared in the *British Medical Journal* about the rise of Stalinism in the NHS and despite the assurances of the civil servants and politicians about 'openness' and 'accountability' the reforms did little to improve the quality of the service.[4] If doctors were too frightened to talk about patients dying from bad management or a lack of resources, they were hardly likely to talk about patients dying because of a poorly performing colleague.

Mrs Thatcher clearly thought that the best way to sort out macho, self-protective doctors was to pit them against each other, confront them with macho self-protective managers and subject them to untested reform. The NHS is not, however, the most enticing job for the cream of management – one told me 'the money's crap and you spend all day fighting fires' – and despite the huge increase in numbers, many managers were inept or ineffectual.

There were power struggles between doctors and managers, loyal long-term hospital employees such as nurses, porters, cleaners and lab staff were replaced with agency or private staff, purchasers and providers sometimes weren't on speaking terms and – predictably – the money ran out halfway through the year. Surgeons would spend six months working their butts off and the other six twiddling their thumbs.

Hospitals were penalized for being too successful and patients were given treatment not according to clinical need but whether the purchasers could afford to pay. At *Private Eye*, I was sent hundreds of hospital memos offering preferential treatment to patients of NHS fund-holders. Short-term contracts meant that many NHS staff feared for their jobs, that their jobs ceased to be vocations, and that patient expectations soared above what the service could deliver. With these came an epidemic of violence and abuse against NHS staff. Operations were still cancelled at short notice, there were not enough beds or specialist nurses and there was still a crisis every winter.

The promised accountability never arrived. In the battles between managers and doctors, it was often impossible to tell who was on the side of the angels, but if the doctors went for a vote of no confidence, the managers usually lost. On the part of the doctors there was little inclination to sort out the good practice from the bad despite millions set aside for audit. The reforms were less about serving the public and more about personal, professional and institutional survival. The ethos of putting the patients' interests above all others was lost in the mist.

I wrote about these issues in *Private Eye*, and also tried to hammer home the message by standing against health secretary William Waldegrave in Bristol West in the 1992 election. In February and March 1992, I used the *Eye* to publicize health problems in Waldegrave's constituency. Tony and I prepared an election manifesto that contained anonymous quotes from frightened doctors working at the Bristol Royal Infirmary, which showed that the problems were not confined to paediatric heart surgery:

- 'In the last four months, nine-four (adult) patients have been refused a bed on intensive care and 40 per cent have died.'

- 'I've been told not to even operate on patients who might need intensive care afterwards. We gave one patient £4,000 worth of blood products but because there were no ITU beds we couldn't take him to theatre and he died.'

- 'The situation's farcical…there are two patients being ventilated in the recovery room and their relatives are packed in like sardines. It's not a bed shortage, it's the staff – they won't give us the nurses for more than five beds.'

There were many more quotes from GPs complaining about how hard it was to get patients admitted to hospital ('no one wants a sick elderly patient. I tried for four hours to get an admission…') and how quickly they were being discharged ('They turfed an elderly patient out on the day of his hernia operation, even though he lived alone and it was a Saturday. He had a big bleed on the Sunday and I had to send him straight back in.') Junior doctors complained as loudly and as secretively as ever ('I've been told to shut up if I want a reference.')

All these were circulated to the local media. The NHS was the battle-ground for the election but Waldegrave disappeared into the ether. On 23 March 1992, he sent a letter to the editors of regional newspapers saying, 'I write to urge immense caution in the use of individual case histories where the NHS is alleged to have failed a patient. Very many of the individual cases alleged have, on investigation, turned out either to be completely false or heavily distorted.'

In the run-up to the election, I was still researching the allegations about children's heart surgery. I told several local journalists what I knew, and that a tragedy appeared to be unfolding in the health secretary's own constituency. However, those who tried to investigate the allegations before the election came up against a wall of denial.

As I followed up the story, I spoke to several people who worked, or had worked, on the heart surgery unit, including Steve Bolsin. I was as certain as I could be that the information I received was the best available, and that babies undergoing the more difficult procedures had much higher death rates than at units elsewhere in the UK. The process of risk stratification was not fully developed but those I spoke to had worked in other units and said that, even allowing for case-mix, the operations were taking longer than elsewhere and the results were much poorer.

I knew that surgeons doing hernia or hip replacements often didn't have much idea what the results were, but I assumed that any super-specialist centre that was spending millions of pounds doing such difficult surgery would be obliged to have its results independently audited. I imagined these were submitted to the Royal College of Surgeons, GMC and Department of Health as a matter of routine, so they could be compared to other units and any 'significant outlier', that is, a unit identified as doing far worse than the others, sorted out. Surely there was some defined minimal standard that could be identified and foolproof mechanisms to ensure it would be acted on?

The answer was no. Audit information that did exist was considered not fit for public consumption and patients who asked about the chances were just quoted a percentage that may or may not have been a true reflection of the real risk.

For example, the 1998 GMC investigation into Bristol found that some parents were quoted a success rate that was much higher than the individual surgeon's average success rate. Nothing was written down and surgeons and patients differed in their recollections of quoted risks. The defence later put forward of the Bristol unit was that Mr Dhasmana was on a learning curve for new operations and that Mr Wisheart took on the sickest patients and so his results were bound to be poorer. Wisheart said that this average rate was based on harder operations, and so with less-ill children it was acceptable to quote a higher success rate. However, the GMC analysed all the figures at great length and decided this had not been the case.

I had tried to start the debate in *Private Eye* six years before the GMC. I realized that publishing raw data wasn't ideal, but the problem had not been resolved in four years and I wouldn't have sent my children or anyone else's children for complex heart surgery in Bristol. I strongly believed that parents had a right to know as much as I did. That was the theory, but the NHS was (and is) so over-stretched that patients were generally grateful just for a bed and a promise of treatment. And most of them didn't read *Private Eye*.

However, when I discussed it with friends who'd trained there, they refused to believe there could be such a big problem. They had nothing but praise for the dedication of both surgeons. Wisheart joined the Bristol Royal Infirmary (BRI) in 1974. He built the Bristol unit up from scratch, worked round the clock to maintain it, was widely respected by his colleagues and was a gifted communicator.

As one of the managers told me in 1998:

> We knew James' results were worse than average but he took on the sickest children so they were bound to be. Even when the press leaks started to come out, he would stand up in disbelief and say, 'Look what they're writing about me now.' I'm certain the trust board had no doubts about him because, as late as 1995, he was on a short list of two to become the next chief executive. I didn't even begin to doubt him until the GMC verdict came through and even now I find it hard to accept. He was always in the hospital and always working. A picture painted of the hospital at the weekend has his white Volvo in the car park. He worked so bloody hard he used to fall asleep in board meetings.

Falling asleep at work may be a sign of dedication, but it may also be a sign that you've taken on more work than you can competently handle. Wisheart became medical director of the trust and chairman of the hospital management committee – positions with huge management responsibilities – and continued doing some of the hardest operations known to man on babies' hearts the size of a plum. It was a ludicrous situation – rather like trying to fly the plane and hand out the drinks at the same time.

There was also a conflict of interest. When Steve Bolsin couldn't get the trust management to act, he went to the Department of Health to complain. He was referred to the 'three wise men', where, as mentioned earlier, a panel of three doctors considers cases in which a doctor's illness or disability may be a danger to patients. 'My problem was that the person I was complaining about, James Wisheart, was medical director and chair of the hospital medical committee, which meant he himself was two of the three wise men. It was completely inappropriate.'[5]

Bolsin spent six years going through all the right channels, trying to expose the fact that children in Bristol were dying unnecessarily. I met him after the first four years. He was very angry, incredibly stressed and intensely ethical. If ever anyone rammed home to me the obligation to put the patient's interest above all others it was him. No one in the NHS goes to work to do a bad job, but there were clearly problems in the Bristol unit which the trust wasn't addressing and parents weren't being informed about.

The Department of Health had known about the problems in Bristol for at least three years but failed to act. Instead, they announced a system of Charter Marks for superficial performance indicators. The United Bristol Healthcare Trust applied for one, and in May 1992 I wrote:

> Before the Department of Health bestows its mark of excellence on the United Bristol Healthcare Trust, it may wish to ponder the perilous state of its paediatric cardiac surgery. In 1988, the mortality was so high the unit was dubbed 'The Killing Fields'. Despite a long crisis of morale among intensive care staff, the surgeons persistently refuse to publish their mortality rates in a manner comparable to other units. And although Dr Roylance (the chief executive) and the Department of Health are well aware of the problems, they won't recognize them officially.
>
> Recently, the unit failed to provide a paediatric cardiac surgery nurse for post-operative care because it was assumed the baby would not survive the operation. And although Liverpool surgeons have successfully operated on 160 babies with Fallot's tetralogy, a congenital heart abnormality, the Bristol mortality rate is between 20 and 30 per cent. Hardly the stuff of commendations.[6]

After publication, I expected the Department of Health (DoH) or GMC to launch an investigation and the trust to release its audit figures. Instead, the DoH and GMC did nothing. The trust made no comment and no attempt was made to counter the allegations.

Shortly afterwards, the new Health Secretary, Virginia Bottomley, declared that NHS whistle-blowers should be heard and protected. So I decided to draw the Health Secretary's attention in person on 3 July 1992:[7]

> Mrs Bottomley claims that whistle-blowing 'through the correct channels' will get results. Staff at the United Bristol Healthcare Trust have been whistling about the dismal mortality statistics in the paediatric cardiac surgery unit since 1988 (*Eye* 793). And while UBHT's chief executive John Roylance, the Royal College of Surgeons and the NHS Management Executive are well aware of the problem, they seem more concerned with silencing the blowers.

In America, the mortality rate for arterial switch, an operation to connect congenitally transposed arteries from the heart is now 0 per cent. Nearer to home in Birmingham it is 3 per cent. In Bristol, despite the fact that the operation has been performed since 1988, it is 30 per cent. Sadly, consultant cardiologists at the Bristol Children's Hospital continue to refer patients to their surgeons to support the local unit. As a recently retired and very eminent cardiac surgeon in Southampton says; '*Everyone* knows about Bristol.'

Again, no official response. I assumed that Mrs Bottomley had staff whose job it was to monitor the media and that someone would have read it. I also assumed that the Royal Colleges, DoH, GMC, district health authority, regional health authority and UBHT board would now realize that the information was coming from inside the unit and needed urgent investigation. But as one long-serving UBHT manager later told me, 'The *Private Eye* articles were read but dismissed as scandal. We believed James Wisheart. We thought that if they just kept trying, it would all come right in the end.'

Until this point I hadn't mentioned anyone by name as I had no way of proving that the poor results were due to surgical technique rather than, say, the failings of other team members or a lack of resources. But on 9 October 1992 I wrote:

The sorry state of paediatric cardiac surgery at the United Bristol Healthcare Trust (*Eye* 793,797) has been confirmed by an internal audit of the last two years' operations. The results of procedures to correct two congenital abnormalities (tetralogy of Fallot and transposition of the arteries) were especially poor. James Wisheart, chairman of the hospital management committee and medical adviser to the trust board, is required to maintain standards of medical practice at UBHT. Curiously he has not felt it necessary to inform the trust board or the trust's purchasers of these findings. Could it be because he is also associate director of cardiac surgery?[8]

After publication, more silence. It was as if the whole trust was in denial. Parents and former patients began to contact *Private Eye*. People who had had successful heart operations at Bristol wanted to express their gratitude to the staff and felt I was being very unfair. Parents whose children were due to have operations at the unit also wrote and my response was that, although the trust wouldn't comment on which operations were going well and which were not, in their position I would insist on going elsewhere.

I've no idea how many were able to. Despite what the politicians say, freedom of choice has always been a mirage in the NHS. The operations were 'designated procedures', which means that the health authority could have sent the babies and children anywhere in the country without financial penalty. So why didn't they? Perhaps they wanted the kudos of an expert centre on their patch, while UBHT wanted the kudos of providing it. If providers deny they have a problem, and the purchasers are happy to keep putting up the money despite persistent rumours that all is not well, then patients are stuffed.

A member of Avon Health Authority – the purchasers – did ask UBHT's chief executive John Roylance about the *Private Eye* articles and he dismissed them. Avon's health authority didn't take it any further and neither did the GMC.

On 3 July 1998 I met Michael O'Donnell who was, until he resigned in 1996, the longest-serving member of the GMC and who had become chairman of its professional standards committee. For twenty-five years this former GP campaigned for more rigorous and open accountability of doctors to sort out poor performance. He met with little support. A notable exception was Professor Ian Kennedy, now chairman of the current Bristol inquiry, who served on the GMC for many years.

Most GMC members did not want to force doctors to audit their work. 'There may have been many other cases like Bristol,' said O'Donnell, 'but this was unique in that someone had gathered the evidence.' After *Private Eye* published this evidence in 1992, O'Donnell raised the issue at a council meeting and was reassured Wisheart was a good chap. The ineffectuality of the GMC was further highlighted by O'Donnell's observation that: 'Two of the consultants who screened cases for the professional conduct committee were alcoholics. At meetings, one used to disappear into the corner with the bottle of wine meant for us all and reappear shortly afterwards spouting gibberish. It was most embarrassing.'

In retrospect, my attempts at whistle-blowing achieved very little. I wish I had gone direct to the GMC, if only for the record, and I wish I had had the media contacts and experience I have now. I was fooled into believing that, if I repeated my concerns in *Private Eye* often enough, something would be done. Given the number of doctors, managers, civil servants and politicians who were at least aware there might be a problem, I still don't understand why something wasn't.

When I left Bristol at the end of 1992, I was told that the matter was in the hands of the Department of Health and was reassured it would be sorted. The operations continued until 1995 because, as a DoH official told the GMC inquiry, even the health secretary would have difficulties intervening to override a trust's decision to let surgery continue. Trusts had been given their independence and there was no stopping them.

Also the patronage system runs deep in medicine and – if you're fond of conspiracy theories – Bristol has its own medical Masonic lodge. Whether this played a part in the cover-up is impossible to say, but there was certainly a lack of insight amongst consultants, intense loyalty between friends, financial pressure on an institution from a market system and an inability or unwillingness of the hospital management to tackle the problem.

There was no help from outside bodies. The GMC, BMA, Royal Colleges, district and regional health authorities and Department of Health evaded responsibility, either ignoring the facts, passing the buck or hoping the problem would sort itself out.

But above all the problem was a lack of values. Doctors are human, we regulate each other in private, we have a human capacity for self-delusion and sometimes we put the interests of ourselves, the profession and the institution above that of the patients.

Perhaps the biggest mistake was to allow paediatric heart surgery to start in Bristol at all. It didn't have a specialist paediatric surgeon, it wasn't a specialist unit, it didn't get enough referrals and when it did, the surgery and intensive care unit were on split sites.

At the time, my hunch that the problem was widely known in the medical community was reinforced through my experiences as a comedian. *Struck Off and Die* were doing a lot of after-dinner cabarets to medical audiences, performing at the Edinburgh fringe, at the Bristol Old Vic and for Radio 4 as well as hosting the Hospital Doctor of the Year Awards in front of the cream of the medical establishment.

On these occasions, we'd talk about the lack of accountability of doctors, and how there was a surgical unit in the South West of England where the mortality rates were so high it was known to staff as the Killing Fields and the Departure Lounge. It even appeared on a Radio 4 CD (*Struck Off and Die*) recorded in 1993. Everybody laughed. We didn't name the unit but sometimes doctors in the specialty would come up to us afterwards and correctly identify it. Occasionally they would identify another unit, which was equally worrying. But it was clear that numerous cardiac surgeons, cardiologists and anaesthetists knew about Bristol well before the GMC acted.

On 23 November 1998, I gave an after-dinner speech to a large group of cardiologists. My first question was: 'Have you ever worked with a doctor whose technique was so bad, he (or she) had a nickname to prove it?' Virtually everyone in the room had. There were Choppers and Shakers and Hackers and Butchers and Bleeders and Squirters and Fumblers. One in every hospital, and lots of gruesome anecdotes to go with them. Next question: 'How many of you actually reported your concerns to the GMC?' No volunteers. Final question: 'My Mum needs a heart bypass. Could you give me the names of any surgeons you wouldn't send your own mother to?' Again, silence.

On 20 June 1997 I gave an after-dinner speech in Cambridge for the Association of Cardiothoracic Anaesthetists. It was clear that many of them knew what had been going on in Bristol. Some spoke openly of the difficulties; others spoke of Steve Bolsin as a hero and a friend, but none saw it as their responsibility to go to the GMC. Bolsin was the one with the evidence. It was all up to him. And he'd been forced out to Australia by then.

The story was finally broken by BBC Bristol on 6 April 1995, months after both surgeons had already stopped operating. One of their final cases was a little boy called Joshua. On the eve of Joshua's operation, nine clinicians got together to discuss whether it should go ahead in view of the vehement opposition expressed by Dr Bolsin, the doubts of Professor Angelini, an adult cardiac surgeon, and the unease of Dr Doyle from the DoH. At no stage did they consider inviting Joshua's parents into the meeting or telling them it had taken place. At 11p.m., Mr Dhasmana gained consent for the operation. At 8a.m. the next morning, he was carrying it out.

The Bristol story was uncovered by BBC West thanks to some excellent investigative work by reporter Mathew Hill. Its transmission relied on the fortuitous loss of a fax from UBHT's lawyers threatening legal action. Had it been found, the story might have been pulled and perhaps have remained buried forever.

The parents of the children who died or were brain damaged were powerless. At present, the only protection patients referred to hospital have in the absence of published audit is the experience and intuition of the doctor referring to the unit. For most operations, a GP refers direct to a named surgeon or a department. Most GPs use a handful of surgeons they believe to be competent because of previous results, rumour or direct experience of having trained with them.

This obviously isn't infallible and doesn't protect against a consultant who goes off the boil or delegates to an unsupervised junior at the bottom of the learning curve. Some GPs refer direct to their friends, some go for the surgeon with the shortest waiting list and some refer to 'any othopod'. GPs are supposed to be gate-keepers and as such we have a responsibility to select a good consultant for our patients. But without the information on which to make that choice, there's a lot of guesswork involved.

It's clear that some referring doctors had been avoiding the Bristol unit for more than ten years. BBC's *Panorama* programme found that as early as 1984 doctors in Plymouth were bypassing Bristol and referring difficult cases to Professor George Sutherland in Southampton. And I've already cited consultants in London who had noticed abnormal referral patterns coming out of the South-west and South Wales in the mid-1980s, with difficult cases referred direct to them.

So why were any difficult cases sent there? Catherine Hawkins, chief executive of the South-west region from 1984–92 told BBC News West that although some cardiologists in the region were reluctant to refer to Bristol, there was pressure on the district health authority from Whitehall, namely the Department of Health, to build up the service. Despite their concerns, cardiologists may have continued to refer to Bristol to support the local unit.

When the public inquiry hears evidence, there are three simple questions for all those who are summoned:

- What did you know?

- When did you know it?

- What action did you take?

My guess is that the answers will expose complicity at all levels – trust, health authority, Royal College, GMC and DoH – and reinforce the need for open audit and a sea change in the self-protective and secretive medical culture. As for what really happened in Bristol, Dr Bolsin believes that the GMC have so far only accounted for a quarter of the unnecessary deaths and that there was a decade of unacceptable practice. 'It's going to be horrible, but it's only when the full roll of accountability has been read that I will consider this disastrous affair has concluded.'[9]

There is, however, a strong counterview in Bristol, from those not happy to accept the findings of the GMC's investigation. Wisheart and Dhasmana's supporters believe that they have been fall guys for a much wider problem, which is true. Their work has certainly been scrutinized more than any other surgeon's in the history of the GMC, and others may have got away with worse results.

They also claim that the GMC failed to accept that Wisheart took on the sickest patients, and point out that the operations in question represented only a small proportion of each surgeon's work. If you divide any doctor's work into small subgroups, you are bound to find one with disappointing results. Finally, as no one had defined a minimal level of competence for the surgical procedures or produced guidelines for when to stop, their only error was a debatable one of judgement in deciding to carry on, decisions that were shared with the whole team.

While I have sympathy with some of those views, the point remains that serious deficiencies in the results of certain operations were repeatedly brought to the surgeons' attention. An ophthalmologist told me: 'You can feel it in your bones when you shouldn't be doing something. You just know. I've stopped doing operations for ptosis (drooping eyelid) because I don't do enough to trust myself to get it right.' A London cardiologist told me that he stopped doing mitral valvuloplasties (to open the valve between the left chambers of the heart) because 'they are so rarely needed there simply is no excuse for not centralizing the service to a few centres. I send mine to Scotland.'

Such insight is commendable, but not universal. Several of the other cardiologists in the same department in London were dabbling with complex 'one a year' procedures and achieving poor results. This has been a recurring theme on *Trust Me (I'm a Doctor)* and is explored in the next chapter. As for Wisheart and Dhasmana, they clearly recognized that they had problems. Dhasmana went for brief courses of retraining and Wisheart repeatedly asked the trust to employ a specialist paediatric cardiac surgeon to take over the work. But still he carried on.

Perhaps to do such technically and emotionally demanding surgery you need such self-belief and confidence in your ability that it becomes hard to analyse your problems with detachment. Again, this only emphasizes the case for independent audit and strong management. In Bristol, there seemed to be as a failure of management as much as anything else.

Wisheart voluntarily stopped operating in 1996. An external assessment of his adult surgery between January 1993 and September 1995 found that his thirty-day death rate for lower risk arterial bypass operations was 12.2 per cent against an average of other consultants of 2.6 per cent. When it came to all coronary artery bypass operations, Wisheart's death rates were 13.4 per cent, compared to the average of 4.1 per cent. For all surgical cases combined, the rates were 13.6 per cent and 5.9 per cent respectively. He was described by the auditors as 'a higher risk surgeon' with a performance that 'appeared to be significantly poorer than the others'. It was recommended that he should not resume operating.

Some doctors I've spoken were surprised that the GMC found either doctor guilty. The dedication and commitment of these two surgeons was never in doubt; their downfall was that their work was being closely audited by a colleague, and that these results were made public.

In the GMC judgement they were found to be incompetent only in making the wrong decisions to operate. There was no direct criticism of their technical expertise or clinical competence, just that they failed adequately to establish the cause of their poor results before continuing. Towards the end of his career, Wisheart was clearly a below average surgeon but if you construct a league table of surgeons half of them will, by definition, be below average. What matters is that all are above an accepted minimal standard yet to be defined. As one of many grateful adult patients who were successfully operated on by Wisheart put it: 'I was just glad I didn't get Killer.'

Ironically, or rather because of all the scrutiny, the new heart surgery team in Bristol is now all on one site and showing the rest of the country how it should be done. Not only are their independently audited mortality figures better than the national average, but they have made them freely available to the public through leaflets and an Internet site. This freedom of accurate information is the only way to restore public confidence. For the first time since moving to Bristol, I'd allow my children to have heart surgery there.

As well as protecting patients, we have to support doctors too. Paediatric cardiac surgeons do the hardest work imaginable and can never get away from it. Ash Pawade, the specialist paediatric surgeon who took over at Bristol in May 1995, has been on twenty-four hour call every day for over three years. How long can any human do that before burning out? Duncan Walker, a heart surgeon in Leeds, was suspended from operating in July 1996 when aged 53. In an interview in *Hospital Doctor*, he realized he no longer had the precision and stamina for paediatric surgery. 'Generally speaking, you are at your peak in your early 40s and a long way past it at 55... If society gets 20 years out of us at full tilt it has done well.'[10]

Most surgeons who go off the boil have given their lives to the NHS. We need to identify poor performance, but we also need to provide for those who are taken out of the operating theatre. Most have a lot to offer in terms of teaching, research and management. As a doctor, recognizing your limitations is tough, but it must always be OK to say, 'I shouldn't be doing this any more.' That deserves respect and reward as much as anything.

4 | TRUST ME, I'M A DOCTOR

"

'Medicine used to be simple, ineffective and relatively safe. It is now complex, effective and potentially dangerous. The mystical authority of the doctor used to be essential for practice. Now we need to be open and work in partnership with our colleagues in health care and with our patients.'

Sir Cyril Chantler, Dean of the United Medical and Dental Schools of Guy's, St Thomas's and King's College Hospitals, October 1998

"

The tragedy of Bristol reinforces just how secretive, powerful and unaccountable doctors are. But Bristol is only the tip of a particularly nasty iceberg.

Rodney Ledward, a Kent gynaecologist, currently operating in Saudi Arabia, was recently struck off after being found responsible for a series of blunders. Gordon Stirrat, Professor of Obstetrics and Gynaecology at the University of Bristol, was Ledward's senior registrar in London when he was a senior house officer. As Stirrat said in supporting a debate on more openness in medicine: 'He was a cowboy even then. The worst I've ever come across in my career. We tried to get him to give up but whoever gave him good references and supported his consultant appointment perjured their soul to the Devil and will carry their consciences to the grave.'[1]

Ledward got away with it for so long because no one was really looking at his results, or if they were they weren't saying. I recently met an SHO who was worried about her consultant. 'From what I've seen of his operating, I wouldn't let him anywhere near my family. But no audit is done so I've got no proof. And after what happened to Steve Bolsin, I'm hardly going to start auditing him in secret.'

My belief that the problems of Bristol are a mirror for what's going on in the rest of the NHS, and private medicine, has been reinforced since we started filming *Trust Me (I'm a Doctor)* in 1996.

Surgeons tend to receive a disproportionate amount of scrutiny in these programmes, partly because their failures tend to be more catastrophic and also because the outcome of what they do is more clearly defined. Hence the gulf between those doing it well and those doing it badly is often clear.

SPECIALISTS DO IT BETTER

One necessity brought about by the small number of doctors in the UK has been the development of the general surgeon, who did a bit of everything. However, as treatments have become more complex, specialist teams have developed for individual operations and, as you might expect, they tend to get better results. For common illnesses and operations (such as strokes and hip replacements) we need lots of specialist centres but for rare conditions requiring complex surgery, there is simply no excuse for not localizing them to a few centres where patients can be guaranteed a good standard of care. But this doesn't always happen and you may have to fight to get the treatment you deserve.

RARE OPERATIONS

Cleft Palate Repair

Cleft lip or palate is usually caused by a failure of the fusion process of the lip, palate and mouth early on in the womb. Around one in 700 babies are born with the deformity and the surgery to correct it can either make or mar a child's life. Unfortunately, in the UK there's no guarantee you'll be offered a specialist team.

The importance of getting the first operation right was first highlighted by a retrospective study, published in 1992, which looked at patients operated on in the late 1970s in London, north-west England, Norway, Denmark and the Netherlands.[2] The two British centres had easily the worst results, with a staggering 48 per cent of patients in the north-west having 'surgically induced growth disturbance of such severity that major maxillofacial surgery would be required in the late teens to correct the damage'. In other words nearly half the British children had to have their jaws broken and surgically re-constructed as teenagers because their early surgery was inadequate.

Simon Whyte was one of the unlucky ones. He had nine major operations in his childhood to correct a cleft lip and palate. He and his mother Gail particularly remember the operation he underwent when he was seventeen:[3]

SIMON WHYTE: It involved breaking the upper jaw on both sides, advancing the jaw so that the bite came into a normal line, taking some bone from my left hip, and grafting that into the gap that they'd created at the fracture site. And then welding the whole lot into place with plates so that it was fixed and rigid and the bones could grow together again.

GAIL WHYTE: I don't think I really appreciated what was going to be involved: seven hours in theatre, intensive care for twenty-four hours...wires and tubes all over the place...

SIMON: I always remember I had a gap in my teeth, and I could fit a straw through this gap and that was the only way I could eat and I had a lamb casserole and strawberries... We had strawberries coming out of our ears... But I lost half a stone in six days.

GAIL: When we eventually got him home...I think Simon really wondered whether it had all been worth it.

Professor William Shaw of the University Dental Hospital of Manchester was part of the team who treated Simon in his teens. Surgery was necessary to correct the gross misalignment of Simon's teeth. Four titanium plates were inserted to hold his jaw in its new position. Professor Shaw believes such major re-constructive surgery would not have been necessary if the operation had been done properly in the first place. 'In a way it signals a failure of the early surgery that was done when Simon was a baby. The more children that have to have this operation, the more it's an indication that something's not right with the surgery that they've had.' I asked why the initial surgery was being done so badly. 'We found that there were something like fifty-seven different centres where cleft lip and palate treatment was done and that I seem to recall that the majority of surgeons did fewer than five lip or five palate operations in any year. I believe that's too few.'

You might wonder why so many inexperienced surgeons go on doing these operations on the delicate faces of young babies when their results are so poor. One reason is that without follow-up and audit they never find out how bad they are. And there is nothing to stop them. In 1996, the Royal College of Surgeons issued a document laying down minimum standards: it recommended that all cleft lip and palate babies be treated at specialist centres, where surgeons perform at least thirty of these operations each year. A recurring theme is that surgeons can easily flout guidelines from their Royal College if they want to. They are not obligatory, and those not following the guidelines are not obliged to show their results are as good as at specialist centres.

Professor Brian Summerlad is a specialist who performs around a hundred cleft lip and palate repairs a year and gets excellent results. He says, 'It's crucial that you get things absolutely right because if we just get the lining up of the margin of the lip, say, half a millimetre wrong, in a baby of this size it's going to be 2mm wrong by the time this baby's an adult and that of course will be a very obvious problem.'

Summerlad is also keen to stress the importance of a specialist team in getting good results: 'I'm fortunate to have orthodontists, speech and language therapists, paediatricians, ear, nose and throat surgeons, who are actively involved in the teams with me. We discuss the problems, we discuss the cases, we review our results and I think that's the kind of atmosphere that you need to improve expertise.'

So why do surgeons without the expertise or support team carry on doing these operations? Summerlad places the blame in part on the Trusts. 'The finances of the Health Service are such that there are advantages for the Trusts to try and carry out the service locally themselves, or at least in the short term. Of course in the long term it may involve a lot of secondary surgery and in fact end up more expensive but people don't take that long-term view.'

Both Summerlad and Shaw believe that these operations should be restricted to ten centres 'with teams that are very tightly composed of specialists who make this a major part of their professional lives'. In 1997 there were fifty-seven centres doing this operation and it is unlikely that anything much has changed.

In 1998, the Clinical Standards Advisory Group (CSAG), an independent source of expert advice for UK Health Ministers, published its report on services for children with cleft lip and palate. Professor Shaw led the research team. After investigating 574 children who had undergone cleft repair in Britain, they found that 40 per cent had poor dental bite, less than a third had a good lip appearance at the age of twelve and fewer than half could speak with normal intelligibility at that age.

The CSAG stated that of the fifty-seven centres carrying out the operation, only six to eight provided good to excellent care and the overall results were five to twelve times poorer than in the six European centres examined. The key factor causing poor training and poor results from 'specialists' [sic] doing one or two operations a year was 'competition between plastic and maxillo-facial surgeons'. Consultants were carrying out petty professional turf wars to the detriment of patients.

This report also found that not only are many surgeons continuing to perform operations they are not competent to do, but that they are failing to keep adequate records or perform proper audit. Only in the area of alveolar bone grafting is there enough information to compare the two specialties. The results are not pretty. Fifty per cent of cases carried out by plastic surgeons failed compared to 32 per cent done by maxillo-facial surgeons. An important factor keeping this appalling situation going is the desire of trust managers to do the operations locally, cheaply, occasionally and badly, rather than refer to a more expensive super-specialist centre.

Whether plastic and maxillo-facial surgeons can bury the hatchet and work in teams for the good of their patients remains to be seen. At least two members of the CSAG appear not to see eye to eye. John Williams, dean of the faculty of dental surgery, described the findings as 'appalling' and added, 'Cleft palate (repair) is part of the training requirements for plastic surgeons. This is quite clearly wrong as it's the only operation they do in the mouth. So when they do one, their expertise is less than adequate.' But fellow CSAG member and plastic surgeon Roy Sanders countered with, 'We've been operating on lips and palates and reconstructing tongues for years. It's plastic surgery that has developed all the processes for reconstruction.' Some surgeons in each specialty are very good at the operation; many aren't.

The CSAG audit is anonymous and does not name poorly performing centres. You are just left to assume the medical profession will sort the problems out in private. In *Private Eye* I named some of the 'low volume' non-specialist units from whom health authorities were purchasing the operation: Exeter, City Hospital Birmingham, Stoke, Wexham Park, Falkirk, Wrexham, Shotley Bridge in Co. Durham, Carlisle and Royal Surrey in Guilford.[4] None of the hospitals challenged the information, although the situation may have changed. For the best, latest advice on your nearest specialist centre contact the Cleft Lip and Palate Association (CLAPA) on 0117 824 8110.

Liver Transplants

Your eighteen-year-old daughter has taken a paracetamol overdose after a split with her boyfriend. She doesn't tell anyone for two days until she develops liver failure together with kidney and lung problems. She needs an urgent liver transplant. Where do you want her to be treated? In an ideal world, the success figures of the seven adult liver transplant units in the UK would be freely available for public inspection. Most would lie within an acceptable range but any centre doing unacceptably badly would be immediately apparent. It would also ensure that appropriate action would be taken.

Comprehensive 'risk stratified' data for liver transplants comparing the seven units were collected in the three years up to 1998 by the Department of Health's National Specialist Commissioning Advisory Group (NSCAG). Given that risk stratification allows for comparisons of like with like, doctors who operate on harder cases aren't unduly penalized. The report was submitted to the DoH in June 1998; at the time of writing it had not been published and when it is it is unlikely that individual centres will be identified.

Given what happened in Bristol, one might expect such fair audit to be made swiftly available. Figures for different centres are available from the UK Transplant Support Service Authority (UKTSSA) but as they are incomplete and not risk stratified they are hence much less useful. A consultant working at a liver transplant centre who heard that, at a meeting of the Liver Advisory Group, the figures had identified a unit performing significantly worse than the others and wanted to avoid 'a Bristol happening in my speciality', asked me to investigate.

My response was that he should report any concerns direct to the GMC, to which he replied, 'I have a family. I don't want to end up like Steve Bolsin.' So I reported his concern to the GMC and tried to investigate myself.

I contacted Professor Paul McMaster, a consultant from Birmingham and member of the Liver Advisory Group. In addition, I spoke at length to Dr Peter Doyle, who oversees the NSCAG audit for the DoH, and sent details of the allegations to the chief executive of the alleged poorly performing trust. The GMC had received no complaints about the liver transplant unit in question and had no idea what the NSCAG figures were. The hospital quoted their UKTSSA figures, which were comparable to other units.

As Dr Peter Doyle put it: 'These previous figures are misleading because, overall, 30 per cent of the information was missing and there was no way of comparing like with like.' So could I see the NSCAG 'risk stratified' figures? No. That is a decision for the Health Secretary. If they are ever released, will individual units be identified? Again, a decision for the Health Secretary. Both Doyle and McMaster were clear about the need for more openness, but they could not give me the information I needed. What I secured from both was a statement that from what they'd seen of the figures, all the units were performing well, and if – after further statistical analysis – a poor unit was identified I could be certain appropriate action would be taken. At the moment, I can't tell you where not to go for a liver transplant only that the Department of Health is ensuring all seven are up to scratch. In secret.

Biliary Atresia
Another example of what happens when you let non-specialists operate is biliary atresia, a rare congenital malformation that prevents bile drainage and causes jaundice in babies. Jaundice in young babies is common, but if it persists beyond two to three weeks it is worth seeking advice to exclude the possiblity of biliary atresia. If children are identified early (within six weeks), they can usually have a complex operation called a Kasai procedure. This takes up to six hours but can improve drainage through the biliary tract. If done well it will reduce the need for a liver transplant or at least postpone it for many years. If done badly the consequences can be disastrous.

In 1985, the *British Medical Journal* published a survey of the results of treatment conducted between 1980 and 1982 on behalf of the British Paediatric Association Gastroenterology Group and the British Association of Paediatric Surgeons. One hundred and fourteen children were identified with biliary atresia, ninety-five had the Kasai operation. They were treated at sixteen different centres by at least sixteen different surgeons, and success was measured according to whether the children were free of jaundice between the ages of ten months to three and a half years. Good results were clearly related to the number of cases operated on in each centre. Only 11 per cent of children treated in centres dealing with one case a year were free of jaundice compared with 29 per cent at centres treating two to five cases a year and 45 per cent at King's College Hospital, London – the only centre to treat more than five cases a year.[5]

The paper deduced that this alarming variability in results was 'probably' due to 'the experience of the surgeon and the standard of perioperative care'. It concluded that the outlook for these children would be improved if 'treatment was concentrated in a few centres, in each of which the vast majority of operations are done by one surgeon'. You might imagine it has all been sorted out. However, the British Paediatric Surveillance Unit two-year survey for 1993–5 was published in *Private Eye*.[6] It revealed that fifteen centres were still doing the Kasai operation and that although the overall success rates have improved, the same depressing variability exists. And in 1995 the DoH, after taking specialist advice, decided to 'de-designate' the procedure, designation meaning that a health authority can refer patients to any specialist centre in the country without having to pay for it. So the pressure is on to operate in-house.

The Kasai operation can fail even at the best centres, but with the close monitoring of a specialist team, this can be picked up quickly and the child referred for liver transplant. On *Trust Me* we featured the tragic story of Victoria Iddon. She not only had a failed operation at a non-specialist centre but the failure went unnoticed for five months, during which time she put on no weight at all, developed rickets from Vitamin D deficiency and was so jaundiced her hair was 'bilirubin yellow'. By the time she arrived at the specialist centre in Birmingham, she was too frail for a liver transplant and died shortly afterwards.[7]

In August 1998, I reported my concerns to the General Medical Council, whose job it is to regulate medical practice. As yet, I've had no reply. On 27 November 1998 Catherine Arkley, chief executive of the Children's Liver Foundation, sent letters to the Royal College of Surgeons, the Royal College of Paediatrics and Child Health and the British Association of Paedriatric Surgeons. A month on, she too has had no reply.

Mrs Arkley also sent a letter to Dr Peter Doyle, medical secretary of the Department of Health's National Specialist Commissioning Advisory Group demanding that action be taken to make treatment in specialist centres mandatory. The reply? 'NSCAG is not in a position to make decisions about service delivery without the agreement of the relevant professional bodies.' Meanwhile, babies die or suffer unnecessary liver transplantation.

The average success rates for the two units doing more than five operations a year (King's and Birmingham Children's) is 64 per cent, those doing two to five is 54 per cent and those doing one a year is 17 per cent. It is perhaps unfair to lump all centres together like this (Leeds also gets excellent results at 77 per cent), but it is clear that the nine centres that do only one operation a year achieve especially poor results. Clearly surgeons who are doing this operation on rare occasions should be stopped. But how?

One way would be for parents to be given the real figures. The downfall of the surgeons in Bristol was not just their poor performance, but that they had quoted parents survival rates for operations that were far better than their own figures. Perhaps, similarly, parents of children with biliary atresia treated at the 'one a year' centres are not always being told that the average success rate is 17 per cent, compared with 64 per cent elsewhere?

Risk management studies in industry have shown that 'unfamiliarity with the task' increases the risk of a procedure by a factor of seventeen, whereas monotony and boredom increase it by only 1.1.[8] The Kasai procedure is only carried out about fifty times a year, so there simply is no excuse for not centralizing it to a few specialist centres which can prove they do it well.

COMMON TREATMENTS

I've concentrated on comparatively rare procedures – child heart surgery, cleft lip repair, liver transplants or the Kasai operation – because these, at least, have had some sort of audit. Being rare, they should be done in specialist centres of proven ability. But what about more common operations? Because of the numbers involved, they have to be done in more units. What do we know about them?

The little research that has been done suggests that, as with rare operations, centralizing the more difficult common operations to fewer centres gets better results. For example, centres doing more than 100–200 coronary artery bypass grafts a year have lower hospital death rates.[9]

Cancer

An observational study of the survival of 3,786 patients with breast cancer treated in the west of Scotland between January 1980 and June 1988 found that, after risk stratification adjustments, 16 per cent more of the women treated at a specialist breast cancer unit were alive after ten years than those who'd been treated by non-specialists.[10] In this study, a specialist was defined as a surgeon with a special interest in breast cancer who works in a dedicated breast clinic with a defined association with pathologists and oncologists, who organizes and facilitates clinical trials and keeps a separate record of all patients in their care.

As Professor Karol Sikora of Hammersmith Hospital explained: 'To get the best possible care, to get the best possible results, to have the best possible chance of surviving you have to make sure that all the expertise is given to you; you can only get that if you see someone that's dealing with a large number of patients with cancer and preferably part of a team that's dealing with specific cancer such as that of the breast or the lung.'[11]

Unfortunately, one in every four patients is still being treated by general surgeons in non-specialist units who see too few of any one type of cancer to be really expert and don't have the necessary team support. One patient, Linda James, was operated on by a surgeon who had limited experience of breast cancer: 'When I woke up from the anaesthetic I investigated underneath the plasters and bandages and I found that the lump that I'd gone in to have removed was still there. I was panic struck. I thought, they've opened me up and they've found something terrible and they've closed me up again.'

Fortunately, that was not the case, they had simply missed the lump. No longer confident she was in the best hands Linda asked around and discovered by accident that there was a specialist cancer unit nearby. She insisted on being treated there, and treatment was successful. Others are not so lucky, and it angers Professor Sikora: 'It's very disheartening for me as a professional to know that we have the skill in this country to treat people very effectively and yet fifteen thousand people or more are dying each year because they're not getting the best possible cancer care.'

Cancer care in the UK has been under review since a report in 1995 (*A Policy Framework for Commissioning Cancer Services*) which was headed by the then chief medical officer, Kenneth Calman, recommended a reorganization into specialist units. This followed research that UK survival rates lagged behind many countries of comparable economic status (1995 Eurocare study). The aim was to give patients the best possible treatment based on the best available evidence and to continue research into the disease and its psychological repercussions. It should end the lottery of cancer treatment by postcode which plagues many other diseases such as infertility and haemophilia.

However, Professor Sikora is still waiting for uniform, expert care: 'Some areas of Britain have been remarkably successful... In others, hopes have been raised and not fulfilled at all levels leading to demotivation and, on occasion, despair... In general hospitals, if you ask at the inquiry desk for the cancer unit, you usually get a blank stare.'[12]

The problems, according to Professor Sikora, are 'lack of money, inappropriate management and clinicians who are resistant to change'. Cancer care, it seems, will remain patchy for a while yet.

In 1997, the NHS executive published the research evidence for 'improving outcomes in colorectal cancer'. This is the second biggest cancer killer, causing 17,000 deaths a year in England and Wales. It becomes more common with age and often presents symptoms such as bleeding from the rectum or a change of bowel habit.

The survey found large variations in the methods used and the success rates for surgery, and concluded: 'Surgery for rectal cancer should be concentrated in the hands of surgeons who can demonstrate good results, particularly in terms of low recurrence rates. Surgeons should monitor their performance by working closely with histopathologists.' But only 5 per cent of them do and the rest really haven't got a clue how they're doing.

Even when a surgeon meticulously audits his work and proves that new techniques can bring substantial benefits, it can take years for these to become widely used. In the case of one Basingstoke surgeon, Bill Heald, it took fifteen years. Bill Heald pioneered the technique of total mesorectal excision (TME) which involves meticulous removal of the tissues lying circumferentially around the rectum, rather than the traditional process of removing a tumour longitudinally. Recurrence rates, colostomy usage and death are markedly lower in his patients compared to those elsewhere in the UK, and although no randomized controlled trial has been done, population studies in Scandinavia, Holland and Germany strongly reinforce this finding. Heald has revolutionized rectal cancer care outside the UK.

The fact that Heald's genius has been embraced by our European partners but largely ignored in the UK says a lot about the way we practise. Surgical training has not allowed specialization to learn new skills such as TME, preferring to produce general surgeons who can do a bit of everything. Some can, but others are getting alarmingly high recurrence rates for the cancer. Back in 1986, Heald published his own recurrence rates of 2–6 per cent compared to the national average of 35 per cent. His colostomy rates are 15 per cent compared to the average of 45 per cent. And by preserving the nerves of sexual function, his impotence rate is also a third of those using traditional surgery. Indeed, there is more variability in the outcomes for rectal cancer surgery than for any other cancer, so it is vital you get a specialist. Also, UK doctors are perhaps less good at admitting their limitations, abandoning their egos and working in specialist teams. Rectal surgery is a good private breadwinner and it can be difficult persuading a surgeon to give up even when audit shows his limitations.

Stroke

What is the single main cause of disability in the UK? What is the third biggest killer? And what is being done about it? Stroke, stroke and not much. Each year 100,000 people suffer a stroke – that's one every five minutes – when brain tissue dies due to a lack of blood supply. The consequences can be physically, emotionally and economically disasastrous. Each year, 5.8 per cent of the entire NHS/social services budget is spent on treatment, and there is good evidence that patients treated in specialist units do better. Back in 1993, the *Lancet* published an overview of all the randomized controlled trials between 1962 and 1993 comparing specialist stroke management with non-specialist. Patients treated in stroke units were 28 per cent more likely to be alive after four months and 21 per cent more likely to make it to a year. In nine out of ten of the units, the patients also achieved 'functional gains' (i.e. were less disabled after treatment).[13]

In 1997, the *British Medical Journal* published a similar review which found that specialist stroke care reduced the chances of dying or remaining physically dependent by 29 per cent.[14] If all patients had access to such care, over 4,500 lives a year would be saved and another 6,250 patients would regain independence compared to conventional care. There is no systematic increase in the use of resources with such care and there is some evidence that hospital stays may be shorter. There is also the potential for huge savings in that many thousands of patients would not need long-term institutional care nor draw disability benefits, and the burden on carers, who currently put in 3.7 million hours a week, would be much reduced.

The Department of Health has at least recognized that stroke care is a problem, costing £2.3 billion a year with patients occupying 20 per cent of acute hospital beds and 25 per cent of long-term beds. The Government's 'Our Healthier Nation' targets include a reduction in the death rate from heart disease and stroke amongst the under-65s by a third. However, good treatment is largely dependent on isolated enthusiasts, and the government has yet to announce any national implementation for organized stroke care. If such a scheme had been implemented in 1993 when the evidence of benefit was clear, many more thousands of stroke patients would have been alive and free from disability. At present, the care you or your relatives receive is a postcode lottery, with those who make it to a specialist unit almost a third more likely to survive and regain independence.

Electroconvulsive Therapy (ECT)

In November 1998, the Royal College of Psychiatrists published an audit of the provision in England and Wales of electroconvulsive therapy, proved to be effective in treating intractable depression when other methods have failed. Despite two previous audits (the most recent in 1991) and clear Royal College standards, only a third of clinics met them in 1996, when the audit finished. The audit showed that only 16 per cent of consultants were able to attend ECT sessions and supervise their juniors, 41 per cent had outdated machines and two thirds had no clear policies to help guide junior doctors to administer ECT effectively. As a friend of mine put it: 'On my first day as a psychiatry SHO, I was directed to the ECT unit and told to get on with it without any training or supervision at all.'

In Scotland, however, the junior staff receive excellent training, the consultants are present at ECT sessions, EEG (brain wave) monitoring with modern equipment is freely available and an audit of outcomes has revealed that over 70 per cent of patients improve after ECT. How can Scotland succeed where England and Wales are failing? Is it resources (Scotland gets more per head of the population), is it working conditions or are Scottish psychiatrists a more conscientious and patient-serving bunch?

Prostate Surgery

For any operation, however specialized, there is bound to be a range of performance and you can't always have the top man. But can you avoid the bottom man? In December 1994, the audit unit at the Royal College of Surgeons published the National Prostatectomy Audit for 1992–3. Data from 5,316 operations was collected from both the public and private sector in four health regions, with 96 per cent of surgeons agreeing to participate.

The results were commendably thorough except that none of the surgeons were identifiable. From the audit, you can see that surgeon 169 has a death rate of six times the average but you are given no idea who the surgeon is. On *Trust Me*, Donna Bernard asked the late Brendan Devlin from the Royal College of Surgeons why identities had to remain secret:

> BRENDAN DEVLIN: The point is that to get the information we need to establish trust between my outfit and the individual surgeons, and if the individual surgeons were thinking the data was going to be used for a witch hunt or something like that they wouldn't trust us to collate the data. We're more interested in looking at trends and if we named the surgeons I don't think we would get the information out in a sensible way, straight away.
>
> DONNA: But you are aware who they are?
>
> BRENDAN DEVLIN: Yes.
>
> DONNA: So would you go to number 169 for a prostate gland removal?
>
> BRENDAN DEVLIN: Number 169? I'm not sure whether he's a urologist. I would go to a surgeon who does a lot of an operation and does it well, if I was having an operation.
>
> DONNA: Which is fine if you can look them up in the Royal College's secret database, but what about the rest of us?
>
> BRENDAN DEVLIN: We must be more open, I've no doubt at all about that... But unless patients are very skilled at epidemiology so that they can weigh up all the probabilities in a situation it's not worth telling them, in my opinion.[15]

Patients might differ. Einstein believed that nothing was so complex that it couldn't be simply explained and although doctors are not in his league, we should be able to find reliable ways of presenting complex information simply. Crucially, there's evidence that patients are no worse than doctors in understanding the role of probability in health care decisions.[16]

At the moment, doctors are not motivated to gather the information, let alone explain it. It has been done anonymously for relatively few operations but, short of hacking into the Royal College of Surgeons database, we don't know who the poor performers are.

Hips

In *Learning on the Job*, I quoted research in the *Journal of Bone Medicine* which found that hip replacements done by trainees are eleven times more likely to fail early, so needing revision, than those carried out by consultants. I suspect in many cases the operations are being done unsupervised. But what about the artificial hips themselves?

Every year 50,000 British people have a hip replacement. When it works, it is one of the success stories of modern medicine – removing crippling pain and doing wonders for mobility. A good hip, well inserted, should last about fifteen years. However, in 10 per cent of cases they fail much earlier. As orthopaedic surgeon Khalid Drabu told me: 'I've had to revise hips within weeks of them having been put in. In one health authority where they looked at their figures, there was a revision rate at five years of 10 per cent. That's 10 per cent of all hips that had been done had to be re-done within five years.'[17]

Surgeon Sarah Muirhead-Allwood was equally forthright: 'Each year I do between three and four hundred hip replacements. About a half of these are in fact revisions [correcting failures].'

A major reason for failure is the hips themselves. There are more than sixty designs. I asked Chris Bulstrode, Professor of Surgery in Oxford, why we needed so many. He replied: 'Well, I don't think we do. I think the companies manufacturing these things have to bring out new products every year because that's what manufacturing's all about. There are some well-proven designs already on the market and we could stick with those if we liked.'

One patient, John Morland, didn't receive a well-proven hip. So far he's had three hip replacements, the first being the so-called 'ring hip' which failed in under a year. Khalid Drabu showed me an X-ray of one such failure. He said: 'There's quite extensive destruction of the acetabulum or the bony socket in the pelvis. The socket is actually migrated inwards...breaking the inner wall of the socket just here. And it's riding up in the pelvis as well... That is entirely the fault of the prosthesis.'

Mr Drabu doesn't use ring hips, but other surgeons still do. It's what they're used to and they don't want to change. Unfortunately, revisions for failed hip replacements are far from straightforward, as Chris Bulstrode explained: 'It's very difficult to do. Only a few centres do it routinely – you need special equipment, it takes a lot of time, it takes twice as long as an ordinary patient so you're taking up two slots on the operating list that could have been used for a first-time-round hip. There's also an element that the patients get very demoralized.'

Some failures are down to poorly tested new prostheses which manufacturers push hard for surgeons to use. As one anonymous consultant put it: 'Drug companies are not much different from arms manufacturers. They fly us all out to Florida, pamper us, brainwash us and then get us to use their latest fancy prosthesis, whether it works or not. We're all in their pocket.' Do surgeons tell patients that they are trying out new, unproven prostheses? Chris Bulstrode thinks not: 'There's no reason why a surgeon should tell a patient that he's trying a new design. In fact he probably wouldn't, because he wouldn't want to worry the patient. And I think that's a tiny bit unfair actually, on the patient.'

But do patients know when a hip fails? Khalid Drabu says they often suffer in silence: 'The hips can all fall apart. They don't know what their symptoms are, what a failed hip is like. They may have leg pain which they may think is coming from another origin. They think their hip's absolutely fine because the surgeon's replaced their hip. They haven't a clue what's going on.'

According to Mr Drabu, of all the sixty or so prostheses on the market at the moment, 'there are three well-recognized, well-established hip replacements in the UK, which have fairly good, or very good track records, and those are the Charnley, the Stanmoor and the Exeter.' John Charnley created a prosthesis in the 1960s, provided the tools to put it in, trained other surgeons and followed up every single operation. His audit was meticulous so we know that his prosthesis works. Today's orthopaedic surgeons are too busy doing the operations to trace their long-term consequences, but some audit is occurring. In East Surrey, they keep a regional X-ray register of all hip operations to establish which prostheses work well and which do not. At the Nuffield Centre in Oxford, they've used an X-ray technique called RSA which detects minute movements of marker beads inserted at the time of the operation. This can predict which new prostheses are likely to fail far more quickly than conventional X-rays.

However, these audit enthusiasts are very much in the minority. We do not have any obligatory national register of orthopaedic implants as they do in Sweden, so most UK orthopaedic surgeons don't know how well their implants do or which are likely to fail prematurely, such as the 3M Capital hip, about which the Medical Devices Agency (MDA) issued a hazard warning in February 1998.

Concerns were raised in 1997 when surgeons in Nottingham published a paper in the *British Journal of Bone and Joint Surgery*. This found a failure rate of 26 per cent at an average of only two years after insertion. The MDA oversees such devices, but they are not required to undergo long-term clinical trials before use, which is bad news for the 5,000 patients who had a Capital. We also have no early warning system for failures. When a new cement called Boneloc [sic] was found to have a high failure rate in Sweden, it had been used on only fifteen patients. In Britain, it was used on 1,800.

In 1993, a *BMJ* editorial warned the 'fashion trade in joint replacements is costing the health service many millions of pounds each year and, even more important, is causing patients unnecessary pain and distress through early failure of unproved implants'.[18] Today the system of introducing new prostheses is still no more evidence based than the fashion industry.

If you're due to have a hip replacement in the UK your best bet at present is to insist on a proven prosthesis. You can't go wrong with a Charnley or Stanmore, although they are hard to find because they have all been modified. Some modifications are good (such as the Elite) others (such as the Capital) are bad. In the Exeter region, the Exeter hip has good results. If you believe they wouldn't stick any old rubbish in the Queen Mum, she had the Furlong. If a surgeon offers you something else, ask to see a long-term audit of its effectiveness.

Amniocentesis

If you were pregnant, would you want an obstetrician to stick a needle into your womb without knowing where the baby is? It happens every day in the UK. Amniocentesis involves drawing off fluid from around the baby in the womb to diagnose conditions such as Down's syndrome. It is usually performed at 16 weeks and parents are told that the risk of causing miscarriage is between 0.5 per cent and 1 per cent. However, this is a very misleading statistic because it is only a national average. In some hands the risk is lower, in some very much higher. An unpublished audit at a centre in Wales found a miscarriage rate of 4 per cent – that's at least eight times worse than the best centres.

A successful amniocentesis depends on the needle reaching the amniotic fluid in the womb without hitting the baby. For more than fifteen years, ultrasound equipment has allowed continuous monitoring so that the needle tip is always in view as well as the placenta and the baby, which has a habit of moving round. It requires training and considerable skill to operate the ultrasound equipment and guide the needle at the same time and some obstetricians (junior and senior) have neither. But they do amniocentesis anyway, because no one checks up on them.

As foetal ultrasonographer Sally Hill explained:

> I think there's very little quality control of amniocentesis procedures in centres themselves, so it's very difficult for women to find out whether or not the person performing their amniocentesis is adequately trained and competent... I am aware of certain centres where they use ultrasound during the amniocentesis procedure, but they're not using it correctly, they do not show the tip of the needle, continuously, during the amniocentesis. If you are not showing the tip of the needle during the procedure, you cannot be sure where the needle is going; it may well be going through the placenta, or it may well hit the baby.[19]

For doctors who have not picked up the skill of continuous ultrasound guidance, they do amniocentesis 'the old way'. They do the ultrasound first, find out where the baby is, put the scanner down, pick up the needle and hope that the baby doesn't move. Often it does. Hitting the baby or the placenta can have equally catastrophic effects. Bad amniocentesis can not only cause miscarriage, but also there is increasing evidence that it could lead to brain damage in surviving infants.

If amniocentesis is done blind, the only way of knowing you're in the right spot is if the syringe is filled with clear amniotic fluid. If it's filled with blood, you've bodged but you get rid of it quickly, hope the parents don't notice and have another go. This is clearly unacceptable. However, it wasn't until 1996 that the Royal College of Obstetricians and Gynaecologists got round to issuing guidelines, stating that amniocentesis must be performed under continuous ultrasound with the tip of the needle always in view.

As we've seen, Royal Colleges carry little clout and some obstetricians just ignore the guidelines. Eric Jauniaux, a foetal medicine expert at London's University College Hospital sees at least one woman a week who has had a failed amniocentesis. Speaking on *Trust Me (I'm a Doctor)*, he said: 'In most of the cases they tell me that there wasn't any ultrasound guidance at the time of the procedure...' 'Does that shock you?' 'Yes.'

Diane and Terry Parnell are amongst the unlucky ones. When Diane went for her amniocentesis, she was scanned before, but not during the procedure. 'The gynaecologist came in and looked at the scan picture that had been taken minutes before…the needle was inserted into my womb and then Terry said, "It's failed, he's going to have to do it again". Same problem, same pain if not more, and blood swirling round in the syringe.'

Dianne did not miscarry, but her daughter Mishka was born blind and deaf, with severe brain damage. There was a large scar on the scalp right over where the damage was. Mishka died when she was two. The hospital admitted the amniocentesis was done badly, but insisted the needle could not have caused Mishka's brain damage. The Parnells turned for help to Oxford pathologist Waney Squier, who has done a study of brain scans and slides taken from Mishka and other children with similar injuries. She has found histological evidence linking developmental damage precisely to the time of the amniocentesis in each case. 'In addition to this, all of the babies that we have examined have had skin marks on the head, suggesting that there was some sort of injury during development.'

The hospital has settled with the Parnells out of court.

Many obstetricians will not acknowledge the huge variation in miscarriage rates or the brain damage that can result from botched amniocentesis. At present, the only way of ensuring it isn't done blind is for patients themselves to do quality checks on doctors. This is difficult. A woman who is already petrified she might have a baby with a congenital abnormality lies on her back and faces an obstetrician with a needle. Is she going to ask if continuous ultrasound guidance is being used?

After doing the story on *Trust Me* I was contacted by two women. One from Manchester had had an amniocentesis done blind by a consultant who didn't speak to her and drew blood on two occasions before giving up. The other woman said that when she found out the consultant she was offered did it blind she insisted on seeing someone else. When she asked the consultant doing it properly why he allowed a colleague in his department to do it blind, he said he wasn't able to comment.

PRIVATE MEDICINE

There's a saying in medicine: 'In the NHS, the patients listen to the doctors but in private practice, the doctors listen to the patients.' I guess that's what you pay for. Instead of being ignored, patronized, stripped naked and yelled at from the end of the bed for five seconds by Dr Nasty, you get the very same Dr Nice mopping your brow for half an hour, feeding you grapes and showing genuine interest. Yes, doctors are as motivated as anyone else by money; notice how cervical smear and child immunization rates shot up when GPs were given target payments.

In the private sector you can have your own room with the Chablis on ice, the on-call chef and as many pillows as you like. You can also choose your operation, your consultant and the date of your admission. However, before you rush off your premiums, here's a small caveat. Private hospitals are not the best places to be in an emergency. In my youth, I worked in one private hospital where the cardiac arrest trolley consisted of a bottle of port and the death certificate book. The protocol was that if critically ill patients were spotted in time, they should be transferred to the nearest NHS intensive care unit. But it's hard to hit the help button when you're critically ill and most of the deaths occurred very privately indeed.

Private hospitals do now have resuscitation equipment and a few even have their own intensive care units – but not always the staff to use them. Surgeons insist on doing major operations in isolated Georgian buildings and then going home for dinner, leaving a single inexperienced junior doctor and three agency nurses to cover the entire hospital. A few years ago I met a New Zealander who was that doctor, and was horrified to find that when one patient started to choke after a neck operation, no one knew how to intubate her. She died well before her consultant was out of his pyjamas.

Such deaths are rare, but Action for Victims of Medical Accidents has identified a disproportionate number of the claims it deals with coming out of the private sector. Key factors are the lack of emergency equipment and medical expertise. As BUPA's medical director, Dr Andrew Vallance-Owen, admitted in the journal *Clinical Risk*, 'It is the case that private practice offers fewer of the safeguards and supports that help to minimize adverse events and reduce patient risk in the public sector.'

I have no problem with people going private provided they're given all the information that allows them to make an informed choice. Some surgeons do major operations in private hospitals without emergency facilities or support, and patients should be aware of this risk. The notion that private patients are all fit and upper middle class is misguided. I know frail, elderly patients who've used up their life savings out of desperation to get a hip replaced or a cataract done. I also know of similar patients having NHS operations done in private hospitals as part of the waiting list initiatives. This might seem like a sensible use of resources, but the sicker the patient, the higher the risk of the operation and the less you want to recuperate ten miles from an NHS cardiac arrest team.

Because of the financial incentive to investigate or operate, patients may either be given unnecessary tests or treatments or, just as alarming, be operated on by surgeons with no expertise in that particular area. In a discussion of the Bristol tragedy in the letters page of the *BMJ* Beverley Webb, chairman of the medical advisory committee at Pinehill Hospital, Hitchin, Hertfordshire wrote:

> What does one do if a colleague who is not an orthopaedic surgeon or hand surgeon operates on Dupuytren's contractures, or a colleague who is not a plastic surgeon performs breast reductions, or a colleague who is not a gynaecologist inappropriately operates on genital prolapse? What do you do if a colleague always finds something to operate on no matter what the patient is referred with? And what do you say to the anaesthetist who always puts in a regional block as well as giving a general anaesthetic in order to bump up the fee? ... All of these examples are observed every week by all of us who have our eyes open. Worse, they are obvious to our nursing and paramedical colleagues, who wonder why we are doing nothing to correct these anomalies... It is therefore urgent that we put our own house in order and do not lose the impetus for change that the Bristol case has produced.[20]

Anyone can set up a private cosmetic surgery clinic anywhere, call themselves a consultant, advertise for patients and even operate, provided they don't pretend to be a doctor.

The GMC binds doctors to 'only perform treatments they are competent in' but this is openly flouted both in the NHS and private medicine. There are no set minimum training levels for doctors who do cosmetic surgery, so surgeons can and do transfer their skills from other specialties. It's a big risk – in surgery, familiarity with the task is vital.

In October 1997, *Health Which?* published an excellent exposé of cosmetic surgery. Two actresses were sent under cover to seven clinics to request liposuction and a breast reduction. In four out of the seven clinics, they didn't get to see a surgeon at the initial consultation and details of the operation were often skipped over to clinch a sale. The worst offenders were in Harley Street.

At West One Clinic, the actresses saw 'consultants' who were in a medical setting but had no medical training at all. They had to press these consultants for information about possible risks, and what came back was very vague. Breast reduction, a three-hour operation with a three-month recovery, was described thus; '…it is not a major operation…not major surgery…there's no more risk than with any surgery'. The two surgeons 'are very good with boobs…they're doing my wife's in the summer'. Both women had to make a decision and pay a deposit before they would be given access to a surgeon.

At LST Clinic, the actresses were urged to use a 'skin preparation solution' every day before surgery by the non-medically qualified 'medical consultants'. It cost £80, and was found to contain just antiseptic. As for surgery, when one of the actresses asked for time to think it over, she was asked, 'Why, are you having doubts about this? … It's a pity because I thought you really wanted to do it at the end of the day'. What if it goes wrong? 'It doesn't…it doesn't…this is why it's very popular.' There was no mention of infection, blood clots and loss of feeling.

Quality control may be patchy in the NHS, but in some areas of private medicine it is completely absent. At present anyone can set up as a counsellor or offer pretty much any sort of therapy without any assurance that it works. Your best bet, if you want to go private, is to be even more sceptical and questioning of what is offered to you in the NHS, and perhaps opt for a unit attached to an NHS hospital. You still may have to use the same car park as the rest of us and you might not have such a good view of the rose-garden, but at least you should sleep more safely.

AND FINALLY…

No one knows the true scale of medical incompetence, and the defenders of the *status quo* often say, 'We can't get rid of the incompetent ones because we wouldn't be left with enough surgeons to carry out operations'. I don't agree. Statistically speaking, most variables in a given population have a 'normal' or bell-shaped distribution, so about 80 per cent of doctors would be clustered around the average. Depending on what level of minimal competence is decided on, it's likely that around 10 per cent of doctors will fall far below it. If re-accreditation and audit occurred at regular intervals, the 10 per cent of poor performers would be picked up. With compulsory retraining, most should safely be able to rejoin the NHS workforce. Can we afford to do without those few who are too abysmal to retrain? I hope so.

5|HELP ME, I'M A PATIENT

"

'The odd thing about British doctors, especially the senior ones, is that most of them are very kind to their patients, very friendly, but when you actually listen to what they say, the information transfer is minimal.'

A South African senior registrar working in the UK, November 1998

'There are two great skills in life. Knowing what you do not know and knowing how to find out.'

Clare Rayner, Chair, Patients' Association

'Doctors are set apart. We are a priesthood with our own rites, beliefs, systems of initiation and tribal practices. And we have special powers. The public turns to us in moments of extremity and expects an answer, even a solution. Often we cannot provide it. We cannot defeat death, sickness and pain. Everyone within the priesthood knows its vulnerability. But the public does not know about that vulnerability. They hope we can deliver and we want to. Indeed our privileges depend on being able to. We are thus permanently conflicted: expected and wanting to deliver, but often not able to.'

Richard Smith, Editor, BMJ, *March 1997*

'To a certain extent, we get the doctors we deserve.'

Simon Sinclair, author of Making Doctors (Berg, 1997)

"

No country can afford the highest technological care for all its population and that might not be a bad thing. That is because there is little correlation between the amount of money poured into acute health services and the general health of the population. Professor Chris Bulstrode, an orthopaedic surgeon turned medical teacher, argues that we need fewer doctors, not more.

More doctors just means more illness. If we want a healthier and happier country we should get rid of a lot of doctors.

I cannot have been the only person who was absolutely incensed to discover that when the Berlin wall came down, the military strength of the Eastern Block was an order of magnitude less than we had been had been led to believe. I want to try all the Western generals for lying to the public about how strong the Russians were. These generals have done three things over the last thirty years. They have frightened the hell out of the Russians, they have frightened the hell out of us, and they have stolen a huge amount of money from the budget that could have been used elsewhere. As I was thinking about this, I realized that this is exactly what we as doctors do about health care.

He has a point. Western medicine is excellent in an emergency assuming you get to the right centre; surgery is brilliant for relieving the distress and disability of arthritic hips and knees, cataracts and hernias; and some life-threatening illnesses can be made much less threatening by good medical care. But a range of treatments are carried at huge cost without any real evidence that they are doing much for the public good. Judging the effectiveness of a treatment is complicated, compounded by the problem of the placebo.

NICE BAT, DOCTOR – BUT DOES IT WORK?

'A French doctor had a patient who was convinced he was possessed by the devil. The doctor called in a priest and a surgeon, meanwhile equipping himself with a bag containing a live bat. The patient was told it would take a small operation to cure him. The priest offered up a prayer, and the surgeon made a slight incision in the man's side. Just as the cut was given, the doctor let the bat fly, crying, "Behold, the devil is gone!" The man believed it and was cured.'

An anecdote of Denis Granville, Dean of Durham 1684–91

'I was brought up, as I suppose every physician is, to use placebo, bread pills, water injections and other devices... I used to give them by the bushels...'

Professor Richard Cabot, Harvard Medical School, 1903

'Whatever the rights and wrongs, placebo prescribing is widely practised and, if we admit it to ourselves, so is the habit of prescribing for largely social reasons.'

Dr K Palmer, British GP, 1998

'Take anything that is either nasty, expensive or difficult to obtain, wrap it up in mystery and you have a cure'

Richard Totman, psychologist and medical researcher into the effects of stress and personality on illness

Faith and suggestion have always been at the heart of medicine. If you believe in a treatment and/or a doctor, you will certainly feel better and sometimes get better, even if he's just given you a sugar pill or let a bat out of the bag. This phenomenon, known as the placebo effect, is extraordinarily powerful and versatile.

Tablets containing no active ingredients can, if you swallow the deception, produce noticeable improvements across a whole range of symptoms and illnesses: pain, tiredness, nausea, high blood pressure, angina, asthma, hay fever, headaches, PMT, depression, anxiety, peptic ulcers, high cholesterol, insomnia, hot flushes and social problems. They can even reduce the frequency of epileptic seizures and reverse the effects of powerful drugs.

In 1954, the *Lancet* was less than complimentary about the beneficiaries of placebos. 'For some unintelligent and inadequate patients, life is made easier by a bottle of medicine to comfort their ego... to refuse a placebo to a dying incurable patient may simply be cruel; and to decline to humour an elderly "chronic" brought up on the bottle is hardly within the bounds of possibility.'[1]

This view of the placebo as a mild psychological tonic for the gullible was blown away in 1955 by Henry Beecher, a Harvard medical researcher, who analysed the effect of the placebo in fifteen clinical trials. Regardless of their intelligence, 35.2 per cent of patients experienced therapeutic benefits. As Beecher put it: 'These powerful placebo effects... can produce gross physical changes' which 'include objective changes in the end organ which may exceed those attributable to potent pharmacological action'.[2] In trial after trial, placebos have mimicked, and sometimes matched, the effects of the chemical drugs that they were tested against.

So how do placebos work? No one is quite sure. Part of their effects may be due to the release of endorphins, naturally occurring pain controllers in the body, in response to the conditioned belief that doctors and what they prescribe will make you better.

Placebos can have side-effects too. Any patient entering a clinical trial comparing a new drug with a placebo is warned about the side-effects of the active drug. However, those taking the dummy pill also suffer. In trials of aspirin for heart attack patients, the placebos caused nearly as much indigestion as the aspirin. When the drug reserpine was used in trials to reduce blood pressure, patients were warned that it might cause impotence. It did, but so did the sugar pills.

Further evidence of the placebo's ability to produce tissue changes in the body was provided by a classic experiment using an ultrasound probe to reduce pain and swelling after wisdom tooth extraction.[3] Patients received either real or dummy ultrasound (the probe was not switched on), self-administered or given by the therapist. Neither the patients nor the therapists knew which they were using. There was also a control group of patients who received no therapy at all.

The results were astounding. Compared to the group who received no treatment, the dummy ultrasound, given by a therapist, produced a 35 per cent reduction in facial swelling. This was even higher than the 30 per cent reduction in the real ultrasound group. The effect was greatest when the probe was held still, rather than used to massage the swelling. Patients who used the probe themselves achieved an insignificant reduction in swelling.

It was significant that the effect was greatest when a therapist used the probe because the placebo effect is an amalgamation of all sorts of things: the faith and past experiences of the patient, the complexity of the treatment, the nature of the surroundings, the belief and bedside manner of the therapist, the reduction in anxiety and the capacity of the body to heal itself.

The effect of placebos on individual patients and diseases is not constant but varies according to circumstances. For example, the placebo healing rate for duodenal ulcers in different studies ranges from 20 to 70 per cent.[4] The ability of placebos to relieve the pain of diabetic nerve damage ranges from 0 to 80 per cent[5] and their success in stopping sickness after surgery ranges from 50 to 100 per cent.

How can we maximize the power of the placebo? For *Trust Me* (11 November 1997) I asked volunteers amongst the Group 64 amateur dramatic group in Putney, London, to help test the strength of a fictional drug, Ketofenfobraphen, which was described as 'a powerful new painkiller that works by selectively blocking the effects of prostaglandin 2 alpha.'

I should have stopped there but I was on a roll, going on to say, 'It's been licensed in the USA and Japan for a year, and sales have gone through the roof. In fact, I'd recommend you to buy shares in the company. Its beauty is that it works quickly – usually within ten minutes – although it can occasionally give you a dry mouth and make you feel dizzy. Mind you, it's expensive – seven tablets for £14.99 and they do not taste very nice – but it's the best drug in its class and I use it all the time for my knee. And when the British Lions were on tour in South Africa, they insisted on having some flown out especially...'

The volunteers were randomly assigned to two groups and told they were being given either Ketofenfobraphen or a placebo. In reality both groups received different coloured placebos. Ten minutes after taking them, they were blindfolded to ensure they would not be affected by what others were doing and were asked to submerge a hand in ice. They were asked to withdraw and raise their hand as soon as it got uncomfortably painful. After five minutes, twice as many volunteers who thought they'd taken the painkiller still had their hand in ice compared to the other group. When I asked if anyone had suffered side-effects as a result of taking the 'powerful painkillers' one woman said she had felt faint and dizzy soon after swallowing the pills.

Simply by telling the groups that they were taking a powerful drug, I had managed to improve their tolerance of pain and caused a side-effect. However, the GMC frowns on such deliberate deception and placebos are no longer prescribed openly in the NHS. However, given that 15 per cent of the population are being prescribed antibiotics for illnesses such as the common cold which antibiotics cannot treat, it could be argued that placebo prescribing is alive and flourishing.

The true scale of placebo prescribing is impossible to judge. You can't separate doctors deliberately using drugs as placebos from those who think there's a possibility that a drug might work even if clinical trials say it probably won't. There's also the problem of patients demanding ineffective treatments and the beleaguered doctor giving in. However, doctors often over-estimate a patient's desire for drugs when an explanation would do just as well.

There are also plenty of surgical procedures which the evidence suggests are of little or no overall benefit (such as womb scrapes in young women, grommet insertions, tonsillectomies and wisdom tooth extraction[6]) but which are still widely practised. Many surgeons defend the operations, claiming they are beneficial in carefully selected patients but some of them have been, in effect, placebo surgery. And very powerful it is too.

Deliberate sham surgery is now outlawed, but thirty years ago a group of sceptical surgeons practised just that. At that time it was fashionable to try to relieve the symptoms of angina (chest pain) by tying off the internal mammary artery, an artery which runs close to the heart. The sceptics could not understand how this could possibly help. So they did a trial. They operated on seventeen volunteers with severe angina. Half had their internal mammary artery tied off and half just had their chests split open and sewed up again.[7]

I use the term 'volunteers' loosely, as no one was told they might have a sham operation. During the following six months, five out of the eight who had the artery tied reported being much improved. But so too did five out of the nine 'sham op' patients.

Cutting people open unnecessarily is overkill, but why not bring back the bread pill? Antibiotic prescribing rose by 46 per cent between 1980 and 1991 with an attendant rise in side-effects and resistance[8] and it is estimated that over £1 billion a year is wasted on futile or ineffective treatments. Clearly, coloured bread balls would do much less damage than unnecessary prescriptions of stronger drugs.

Their appearance can also be cleverly tailored to the vagaries of the human psyche. Capsules are more powerful than tablets, especially if they're big, or small, have a bitter taste and a silly name. Colour too is vital: green works best for anxiety, red for pain and yellow for depression. For some inexplicable reason, creams and ointments are strongest in blue or green, elixirs are best in red or brown.

Placebos are regularly used in private practice and on the continent; they could save the NHS a small fortune. As Edzard Ernst, Professor of Complementary Medicine at Exeter University told *Trust Me*: 'Most of my colleagues and myself use placebos in Germany. I also worked in Austria...the climate seems to be a little bit different on the Continent, I believe... In England people are very much against prescribing placebos and I do not quite understand why.'

One answer came from the Group 64 actors. Asked if they would mind being deliberately deceived by their doctors if it meant feeling less pain, they answered with an overwhelming 'yes'. One man said he would deeply resent paying over £6 for chalk.

For those who like a tonic but do not want the doctor to lie to you, there is an 'ethical placebo'. In an American study fifteen psychiatric patients suffering from neurotic symptoms were invited to try a placebo. The doctor's carefully worded request was: 'We feel that a so-called sugar pill may help you. Do you know what a sugar pill is? A sugar pill is a pill with no medicine in it at all. I think this pill will help you as it has helped so many others. Are you willing to try this pill?' Fourteen said yes. Of these, thirteen improved, some a great deal including one previously suicidal patient.[9]

In the UK, the trend has been to dispense with dummy tablets altogether and concentrate on maximizing the placebo effect of doctors by teaching communication skills. In 1985, even the *Lancet* stressed the importance of doctors as human placebos: 'The doctor who fails to have a placebo effect on his patients should become a pathologist or an anaesthetist...in simple English, if the patient does not feel better for your consultation, you are in the wrong game.'[10]

The importance of emotional support and belief applies to all health professionals and complementary therapists. Many of the latter are gifted communicators and have much more time to tap into your mind. But there are limits to the power of the mind to heal the body. The mind may help the body heal benign stomach ulcers or reduce the swelling after tooth extraction, but there's no evidence alone that it can cure cancer. Steer clear of anyone who claims it can.

But if all treatments have a placebo element, how do you know if what's being offered is any more effective than a flying bat?

THE RANDOMIZED CONTROLLED TRIAL

'Drug companies shout from the rooftops that "Fabuloson" made 50 per cent of patients better, but nobody tells us that 30 per cent got better on chalk.'

Dr John Wright, consultant epidemiologist

'A desire to take medicine is perhaps the great feature which distinguishes man from other animals.'

Sir William Osler, Canadian physician (1849–1919)

'Reality is a crutch for people who can't cope with drugs.'

Lily Tomlin, American comedienne

Before the Second World War, decisions about the effectiveness of treatments were largely based on personal experience, rather than objective clinical trials. In 1948, the *BMJ* published the results of the world's first randomized controlled trial into the use of the antibiotic streptomycin in tuberculosis.[11] In such a trial, the new drug's effectiveness is judged on whether it can significantly outperform a placebo using carefully selected volunteer patients split into two random groups.

Neither those giving nor those receiving the drug should know who gets the real thing and who gets the dummy. Some patients, however, are difficult to fool. I once changed a man's tablets to a better brand although it was the same drug, same size, colour, shape, same line across the middle. A few days later he came back and said, 'Doctor, those tablets you gave me, they weren't the same' I asked, 'What do you mean?' 'Well, the first lot sank when I threw them down the toilet and these ones float.'

Testing whether a new surgical technique really works is harder. Placebo surgery is frowned on, although I did hear of a recent trial where microwaves were stuck up patient's anuses and in only half the cases were they turned on. For new surgical procedures, such as keyhole surgery, it is acceptable to compare the new method with an older one or sometimes with non-surgical treatment. Obviously, you can't 'blind' the surgeon to which procedure he's doing and trials of surgery are a test both of the competence and expectations of the surgeon as well as the effectiveness of the procedure. Sometimes they can be hard to separate.

Trials of medical treatments may be more straightforward, but if the disease is not immediately life-threatening the benefits of treatment are likely to be less spectacular and may occur only after a long period of time. In such cases, statistical proof that a treatment works can be hard to achieve. Single small trials rarely prove anything. You either need a single very large trial that you follow up for years or, more commonly, you have to mathematically analyse the results of lots of smaller randomized controlled trials – a procedure known as meta-analysis.

Proving that something does not work is just as important as proving that it does. In 1986 the World Health Organization published a trial showing that anti-oestrogen drugs were of no benefit in treating men with low sperm counts. Yet a recent audit of Scottish urologists found that

80 per cent were prescribing them. The false reassurance of ineffective treatment can mean that couples are left waiting when time is of the essence and they need referral for assisted conception.

Another example is routine breast examinations. GPs are doing them because they believe that routine breast examination is a useful screening test for breast cancer. But as breast cancer specialist Professor Michael Baum points out, the evidence is that they are not:

> If a woman goes to the GP with symptoms unrelated to the breast and there's no question of hormonal treatment and the GP says, 'Well, whilst you're here I'll check your breasts,' she should say politely and firmly, 'No, thank you very much'. If he persists then she's entitled to demand, 'Why do you want to examine my breasts?' and if the GP says, 'Well, I just want to be opportunistic in checking you out as you're passing through,' you should say, 'No, thank you'.

We've known this for some years, so you'd imagine the news had filtered down to GPs and practice nurses. But when Donna Bernard interviewed a random selection of women on *Trust Me*, she found many who had had it and did not like it. 'Well, I went to go the doctor for something or other and he just gave me a breast examination, then and there on the spot, and I just felt very uncomfortable with the whole situation and came away in tears.'

This even happens to women who are doctors. One interviewee commented: 'When I was 16 I went to the doctor for a routine examination and during the examination the doctor examined my breasts and it was only years later, when I was a doctor myself, that it occurred to me at a screening conference that it was completely unnecessary to have a breast examination at that age.'

After the programme went out, women stopped me in the street to talk about it and a secretary in my department told me how it happened to her and to her mother. We also received a letter from a woman who went for a job at one of the Royal Colleges and said she was given an unnecessary breast examination as part of her medical. Shortly afterwards, the Chief Medical Officer issued guidance to all doctors on the inappropriateness of routine breast examinations.

There are hundreds of examples of ineffective treatments still being used and of effective ones being ignored. Many patients who have had heart attacks are not being given aspirin (which helps delay the clotting which causes them), and many patients in heart failure are not on

ACE inhibitor drugs despite strong evidence that both reduce mortality. The truth is that doctors can't keep track of every disease whereas you, as the patient, with relatively few diseases, can easily learn as much if not more than your doctor if only you had access to the information.

Since filming *Trust Me*, I have been impressed with how informed and helpful most health support groups are. Not only do they provide patients with well-written information about what works and where to find a specialist centre, but they also know what it means to be a patient or relative, something often lacking in doctors. Ideally, health groups who hand out balanced accounts of the best available treatments should be hallmarked for identification. For a comprehensive list of such groups see *The Health Address Book* by the Patients' Association, telephone 0171 242 3460.

IS IT WORTH BOTHERING?

'A medical degree is no substitute for clairvoyance.'

George Bernard Shaw

Sewage workers have done more for our health than medicine and the 150th anniversary of the Public Health Act deserved as much, if not more, celebration than the comparatively modest achievements of the NHS. In the last fifty years better health care has contributed three out of the seven years of increased life expectancy and an average of five years of partial or complete relief from the poor quality of life associated with chronic disease.[12] However, by far the strongest predictor of ill health, disability and premature death in this country is poverty.

Back in the NHS, the average benefits of any given treatment can seem rather modest given what you have to go through: for instance, eighteen months of extra life for a coronary artery bypass graft. However, within that average some patients benefit far more than others. In general, the sicker you are, the more you stand to gain from treatment.

Deciding whether to have treatment depends on many things: your beliefs and experiences; whether you have to pay for the prescription; and how the information about risks and benefits is presented to you. If you've had a heart attack or suffer from angina and want to reduce your risk of dying from heart disease, a doctor might recommend a cholesterol drug and leave it at that.

But what if you asked the doctor to put some numbers where his or her mouth is? I suspect the doctor would not have a clue, but with the benefit of the research in front of me, here are just some ways the information could be phrased:

- 'If you take this drug every day for five years, your risk of death will be reduced by nearly 40 per cent.'

- 'If thirty-three people like you take this drug every day for five years, one death will be prevented but I don't know whether it will be yours.'

- 'If you swallow 1,825 tablets of this drug at a rate of one a day for five years and at a prescription cost of £400, your risk of death would fall by 0.9 per cent. The recognized side-effects are muscle damage, headache, abdominal pain, nausea, vomiting, hair loss, anaemia, dizziness, depression, nerve damage, hepatitis, jaundice, pancreatitis and hypersensitivity syndrome.'

Which of the statements is most likely to convince you to take the drug? All the statements are about the same cholesterol-lowering drug, pravastatin, but the first – the relative risk reduction – is the one most quoted in press releases, advertisements and newspaper headlines. Naturally, the drug companies are keen to hype up the benefits and doctors are as gullible about statistics as anyone.

NUMBER NEEDED TO TREAT

The science of medicine is about probability rather than certainty. The chance that you will benefit from any treatment is low, often well below 50 per cent. You can tease out the truth if you ask what the Number Needed to Treat (NNT) is. This means the number of patients who need to be treated over a given period to prevent a specified nasty thing happening to one of them. NNTs are usually much higher than you'd think.

For example, research shows that for every seven children with acute middle ear infection treated with antibiotics, only one will benefit. We can't tell which one, just that your child's odds are one in seven.

If twenty people with a heart attack are treated with a clot-busting drug (aspirin or streptokinase), one person will be alive five weeks later who would not have been if no one had been treated. But we can't tell if it would have been you.

For every 850 middle-aged men (aged 36 to 64) with mildly raised blood pressure taking anti-hypertensive drugs, one stroke will be prevented each year. For elderly hypertensives, the NNT is only thirty-four; that is, the older you are the more you have to gain from treatment because the risk of a stroke is more.

The popular wisdom is that patients do not understand numbers, but the truth is that doctors are as prone as anyone to plucking figures out of the air. John Allen Paulos, an American mathematician, recalls a twenty-minute conversation with a doctor where the doctor stated variously that the procedure he was contemplating had a) 'a one in a million risk associated with it' b) 'was 99 per cent safe' and c) 'usually went quite well'.[13]

Whether you decide on a treatment depends not just on the likelihood that it will benefit you but also on a whole host of factors, ranging from the severity of the illness (i.e. what might happen if you do nothing), the possible side-effects, cost and the need to be in tip-top form for Auntie Beryl's coming out party a week on Tuesday. But knowing the NNT at least gives you the odds on which to hang your beliefs.

If you are interested in finding out more, an ever-growing list of NNTs is provided free on the Internet by Bandolier at http://www.jr2.ox.ac.uk/Bandolier.

SCREENING TESTS

Screening aims to provide an early warning for diseases that allows you to take action to avoid them. Like all of medicine, it's of most benefit to those already at high risk of a disease because of their medical history or inheritance. Screening whole populations is much more hit and miss, and there needs to be strong evidence that it works before we all rush out and get tested. At present, this evidence is lacking for most mass testing (e.g. for cholesterol levels and prostate cancer) and before we introduce any more, we need to learn from what we do already.

Screening for cervical cancer has never been evaluated in a randomized trial although there is good evidence that it is saving perhaps between one and two thousand lives a year in the UK. To save those lives we need to do 3.7 million smears a year on women aged 20 to 65; 250,000 of them will come back abnormal and 50,000 women will be referred for colposcopy. We screen about 4,000 women in order to prevent one death, and for every 250 women with abnormal smears, one life will be saved.

Smears, of course, come in different stages of abnormality. Most mildly abnormal smears stay that way or return to normal. About one in twelve moderately abnormal smears would, if left alone, progress to cancer, and the same is true of about one in three severely abnormal smears. The crucial point is that none of these *are* cancer – it's just that cells have been identified that might, but probably won't, become cancerous if left alone. Continuing with screening or having treatment is the best way to ensure that they won't.

Put like that, cervical screening seems entirely sensible, which I'm sure is why most women go for it. Unfortunately the message that an abnormal smear does not mean cancer doesn't always filter through and some women become profoundly anxious about having cancer when the risk is very small. It could be argued that their lives would have been less stressful if they had not been screened. They certainly should have been given balanced information before they embarked on screening which, after all, is a life-long process.

Screening will never prevent all cervical cancer. Some cancers appear after 'missed' smears – the results of human error, poor management and over-stretched labs. However, most 'failures' are caused by the fact that no test can ever be 100 per cent reliable, and some cancers will always develop in between screening. The other point worth making is that cervical cancer was rare even before screening. Only one in 4,000 women of screening age would develop it anyway. Given this low risk and the inconvenience of smears, I know female doctors, including a gynaecologist, who do not bother to have smears themselves. It is a risk they're happy to live with, even though they advocate screening in others.

One relevant fact is that GPs are paid bonuses to hit smear targets so you may find yourself being pressured into one against your will. Of all the screening programmes, cervical screening is one of the best – in terms of lives saved and horrible illness avoided, and most women who get cancer have not had smears. If you are over 50, for example, and have had regular, normal smears, the chances of your developing cervical cancer are almost zero.

On the other hand, cervical cancer is a rare illness. If your chance of getting it even without screening is very small and if you're the kind of person who may be worried by the much more common abnormal result, it may not be for you. Like all medical decisions, it's more complex than meets the eye.

GETTING INVOLVED WITH DOCTORS

'Remember, there are only four cures in medicine – the patient moves to another area, the patient changes doctor, the patient dies, or you die.'

CG Ellis, Making Dysphoria a Happy Experience *BMJ vol 293 1986 pp 317–8*

'Saved two, killed one... or was it the other way round?'

'Life is a pool of shit, and our job is to direct people to the shallow end.'

Two retiring GPs reflect on fifty years in practice

What do you want from a doctor? Slightly dishonest reassurance or totally honest uncertainty? When I was a trainee GP, I used to disappear behind the curtains or into the toilets with a textbook to swot up on something I'd forgotten or didn't know. Now I just open the book in front of the patient, thinking I'm being disarmingly frank. But what is this doing to my placebo effect? A friend told me about going to see his GP with a skin rash. The GP looked puzzled, took two dermatology picture books down from the shelf and they each looked at one with the GP saying, 'Tell me if you spot anything that looks like it'.

A study by a Southampton GP supported the fact that patients do not like uncertainty.[14] The GP selected 200 patients with sore throat, nasal congestion, cold, giddiness, tiredness and general aches and pains. They were not seriously ill, but he could not be sure what they'd got. He decided to compare the effect of telling them honestly about his uncertainty with a firm diagnosis and promise of recovery. He also wanted to know if adding a placebo prescription made any difference to their recovery. He divided the patients randomly into four groups: A, B, C and D:

- Group A was given a firm diagnosis and a prescription for a drug they were told would certainly make them better

- Group B was given a firm diagnosis and told they required no prescription to get better

- Group C was told, 'I cannot be certain what's the matter with you' and given a prescription with the instructions, 'I'm not sure if the treatment I'll give you will have any effect.'

- Group D was told, 'I cannot be sure what the matter is with you and therefore I will give you no treatment.'

Two weeks later, 64 per cent of those given a deceptively positive consultation were better, compared with 39 per cent of those who were given honest uncertainty. Adding in a prescription made very little difference, presumably because the doctor had already maximized the placebo effect by being so positive. This study has been cited as evidence that doctors should not share too many doubts with patients. Patients don't want to be told the truth about the uncertain nature of their illnesses and are better off with 'beneficent paternalism', an approach doctors have used for more than 3,000 years. In short, the doctor decides what's best for you and, as with the bread pill, a 'minor' deceit is justified if it does you good.

In this study reassurance worked because the illnesses were not life threatening and the patients would have got better in time. Telling people with more serious illnesses that they will definitely get better risks the damage of false reassurance if they don't. It is possible, although harder, for a doctor to be honest and instil confidence. This is more likely to occur if individual patients have some control over how much, or how little, information they're given. In an emergency a patient may not want this; if you're having a heart attack, for example, you may just want something for the pain rather than to be given all the side-effects of diamorphine; but when you're over the worst bit, you should be able to be involved in decisions about treatment.

DO DOCTORS GIVE UNBIASED INFORMATION?

No. This does not necessarily mean the information given is wrong, but rather that the positive side of treatment, or screening, or following what the doctor says tends to be accentuated. This may not be a problem if all goes well, because the doctor has maximized his or her placebo effect. But again it risks the dangers of false hope if the treatment goes wrong. Also, doctors' decisions are not based only on medical factors but may also be biased by your age, sex, ethnic group, social situation or how the doctor judges your quality of life (often wildly wrongly).

Patients often ask a doctor, 'What would you do if it was you/your son/your Auntie Millie?' The answer will be individual, depending as much on the doctor's beliefs and experiences as on the scientific evidence. Doctors in different specialties vary in the choices they would make if they themselves had advanced cancer. When treatments are uncertain or disputed and the outcome unpredictable, they often differ in what they would recommend. Evidence-based medicine should be an international concept, with hard science trumping irrational cultural beliefs every time. But it isn't. If you have a stomach ache, in France you get a suppository, in Germany a health spa, in the United States they cut your stomach open and in Britain they put you on a waiting list.

THE IMPORTANCE OF FEEDBACK

Some doctors are almost idolized for their crass communication or poor technical skills. Very few patients, junior doctors, nurses or students would dare let a consultant know the damage he or she was causing. There's some bullying from the top down and some arse-licking from the bottom up, but rarely is there open, honest exchange.

I was attracted to communication skills training by the importance given to feedback. A key feature of the training is that the simulated patients give constructive feedback to the students about how they felt, whether they had a chance to express their concerns and whether they could understand the information given to them. The actors are now so used to the process that when they see real doctors for real problems, some of them will tell the doctor how they thought he or she handled the consultation.

If doctors and patients really are going to work in partnership, such feedback needs to be commonplace. If you don't tell someone that they have upset you or that you haven't understood a word they've said, they will be likely to repeat the same mistakes every time you see them. On the other hand, many doctors slog their guts out for forty years in the NHS and rarely receive a compliment. Praise is the best motivator, so if your doctor has done something good let him or her know.

You also have a right to a second opinion. You may have to fight for this, but if you've lost faith in whoever is treating you there is little point in persevering. Doctors can't be all things to all people, and you should not let misguided loyalty or the fear of upsetting a doctor get in the way of what's best for you.

PUTTING DOCTORS TO THE TEST

We can't all have the very best doctor and, to repeat an earlier point, if we constructed a league table of GPs or surgical teams half would, by definition, be below average. The NHS also needs to train new doctors and so we can't demand those at the very peak of their learning curves. However, what we should be able to demand is a treatment that's been proven to work and either a doctor who's competent to deliver it, or a doctor who will be closely supervised by one who is.

Competence is a hard thing to define and, as I've said, even senior surgeons will occasionally come up against an operation they have not attempted, or have rarely attempted, before. In some cases, they may rightly feel they have the skills to do it. As Bob Taylor, an ophthalmic surgeon in York, explained:

> There are many operations to correct different types of squint, some of which are much commoner than others. I've published my audit figures for a long series of squint operations but most of them refer to the commoner type. However, if a patient has a rare squint I would feel confident that I could do it because I'm operating in that part of the eye all the time.

So what does he tell his patients? 'If patients or parents ask to see my figures I shown them, and if it's a rare squint I tell them that I haven't done as many but explain why I feel competent to do it.'

This is clearly very different from surgeons attempting occasional operations in areas of the body that they very rarely go near. And, just as importantly, this surgeon is being completely honest and open about his own results and experience. Out of necessity rather than irony, the Bristol Royal Hospital for Sick Children has posted an audit of surgeon Ash Pawade's child heart operations on the Internet (www.ubht.org.uk):

> Over the last three years, Mr Ash Pawade has undertaken 670 cardiac operations, with a total of 22 deaths, giving an overall mortality rate of 3.3 per cent. This rate compares with a national figure of 4.6 per cent. The mortality for open (when cardiopulmonary bypass is required) and closed heart procedures was 3.7 per cent and 1.8 per cent respectively, compared with combined national mortality data of 5.9 per cent and 1.9 per cent. For 1997–98, the mortality rate for all open heart surgery was 4.5

per cent, compared with the most recent national data of 5.2 per cent. The rate for all closed heart operations during this year was 1.7 per cent, just slightly higher than the national comparison of 1.5 per cent. If this closed heart data is broken down into age categories, as undertaken in the national registry, the mortality in all sub-groups is, however, below the national average...

The Bristol unit is the only one I have found that is publishing results of a named surgeon, but there is now a growing number of doctors happy to share their results with patients. Not only do many of the doctors I've interviewed believe in more transparency in medicine, but they actively encourage patients to ask awkward quesitons and seek out better care. As one consultant put it:

As doctors, we all know what sort of questions we'd ask and what sort of treatment we'd want for ourselves and our family. And if it isn't available at the local hospital, we'd insist on going elsewhere. Is it right that patients should be denied that inside information and better service? I don't think so.

The advice is consistent: ask questions. We get plenty of feedback that the message is getting through. Most patients find that doctors view their questions as legitimate rather than awkward, and are happy to provide answers. Some patients complain that the answers are often, 'I don't know', but at least their doctors are being honest (although there is the issue of possibly countering the placebo effect, mentioned earlier).

Some doctors have complained to me that we're making work for them. A plastic surgeon said that after the *Trust Me* programme went out, several of his patients started asking questions about how many operations he does, whether he's part of a specialist unit and what the results are. He may be overworked, but it's a small price to pay if it helps stop the first seventeen years of someone's life being blighted by multiple, major reconstructive surgery.

I cannot stress enough my hope that in the future all this information is freely available to patients in their own homes and GPs in their surgeries, so consultants won't need to spend so much time justifying what they do. But, at present, this information is not available and, even if it were, the quality of care in the NHS is very variable. As the Government document *A First Class Service: Quality in the New NHS* pointed out: 'In one region, amongst thirty-five surgeons, rates of mastectomy for breast cancer varied from nil (meaning all women had breast conservation surgery) to 80 per cent.'

The Government believes that it can improve quality and iron out inequality by imposing reforms from above. We have been inundated with such reforms in the past and they don't appear to have achieved much. Improvements in quality in the NHS are far more likely to come from below, by improving both the standard of medical training and communication between NHS workers and patients.

REASONABLE QUESTIONS FOR ANY DOCTOR

There are many self-help groups and booklets that provide lists of typical questions: for example, the excellent BBC Education *Cancer Guide* recommends that before you have tests and treatment, you might ask:

- What do you think is wrong with me?

- What tests will I need?

- What do the tests involve?

- When will I know the results?

- What treatments are there to choose from?

- What are the risks and benefits of the different options?

- Will the treatment affect my work, study, sex or social life?

- How long will the treatment last?

- How do I know if I'm getting the best treatment?

- Will I be able to look after my family or will I need help?

- Will the treatment affect my fertility?

- Will I be able to drive?

- How can I tell my family and friends?

There is a limit to how much you can absorb when you're worried and ill, and a good centre will provide you with good-quality written information about what to expect and the credentials of the unit. If you're concerned that you may have been referred to a centre that is not up to the mark, you could ask:

- Is this a designated specialist centre?

- How many operations like this do you do?

- What are the results of your audit?

- Has it been published? Was it risk stratified?

For cancer operations
- What is your local recurrence rate?

- What is your five year survival rate?

For any operation
- What is your failure rate?

- What is your wound infection rate?

- How do you compare to the national average?

For a particular surgeon, you might ask:
- Are you a specialist?

- How many of this particular type of operation have you done?

- If a junior surgeon is doing my operation, will he be closely supervised by a specialist?

- What have your results been in the long term ?

- Do you have any published audit you could show me?

- How does it compare to the national average?

For any treatment
Ask about the strength of the evidence supporting its use. There are generally four levels of 'proof', ranging from good (A) to poor (D).

A. Evidence derived from randomized controlled trials

B. Evidence from non-randomized trials or observational studies

C. Professional consensus

D. Personal opinion

In much surgery, the standard of proof is still poor and you have to make decisions based on personal opinion – so the more doctors you see, the more opinions you'll get.

Ask about the Number Needed to Treat (NNT) to prevent whatever it is you're trying to avoid such as death, a heart attack or a stroke. This information gives you the odds of benefiting from the treatment. You can then combine this information with your own beliefs, what will happen if you do nothing and the likelihood of side-effects.

The Number Needed to Harm (NNH) is the number of patients who can have a treatment before one gets a nasty side-effect, and the Number Needed to Screen (NNS) is the number of people who have to have screening to save one life or unpleasant event, such as a case of cervical cancer.

If you can get the hang of asking for specialist centres where large numbers of patients are treated, information about standards, access to audit that shows these standards have been met and guarantees of junior supervision, my guess is that you'll probably get the quality service the Government says everyone is entitled to. And if you ask doctors about the strength of evidence and NNT, you'll start shifting the culture from simplistic, paternalistic reassurance to a meeting between adults.

Part 2

A CONSUMER'S GUIDE TO TREATMENTS

6|YOU ARE WHAT YOU EAT

Pellagra. It sounds like an Italian dish but is actually a very unpleasant disease characterized by diarrhoea, dermatitis and dementia. In other words you get the runs, scaly skin and go mad. At the turn of the century doctors were convinced that pellagra was caused by an infection. In the United States, where this disease had previously been rare, there were huge and totally unexplained outbreaks. Hundreds of people died and no one knew what was causing the epidemic.

Dr Joseph Goldenberg of the US Public Health Service was keen to find out and decided to do an experiment – on himself. He took blood from one of his patients who had a nasty outbreak of pellagra and injected it into his own shoulder. Then he collected phlegm and mucus from the mouth and nose of the patient and rubbed it into his own mouth and nose. At this point this was a disease for which there was no known cure. Nausea, vomiting, bloody diarrhoea, depression, psychosis, scaly skin: these were all things he could look forward to if the experiment worked. It didn't.

Goldenberg obviously decided that he hadn't gone far enough, because three days later he went the whole hog. First he swallowed some sodium bicarbonate to neutralize the acid in his stomach and maximize his chances of getting infected. Then he swallowed, in turn, samples of urine, faeces and skin taken from his obliging if somewhat puzzled patient. Not surprisingly, he got one of the three Ds – diarrhoea – but he didn't develop pellagra. At this point, most people would have decided to give it a rest, but a few days later he was back having another go. This time he managed to persuade a number of friends to join him in once more eating skin, faeces and urine from a pellagra patient. None of them developed pellagra. Goldenberg must have acquired a taste for these items as he repeated this experiment several more times before he finally convinced himself that pellagra was not an infectious disease.

After many years of research it is good to be able to report that he tracked down a cure for pellagra: brewer's yeast. Pellagra, it turns out, is caused by a shortage in the diet of niacin, one of the B vitamins. Once this was understood, the reason for the outbreaks also became clear. At the turn of the century people had changed their eating habits, going from wholemeal grain to fancier and finer ground grain. Unfortunately this process also removed some essential vitamins, including niacin. With niacin added back into the flour, the pellagra epidemic disappeared. For a fuller account of Goldberg's heroics, and that of many other self-experimenters, I recommend the very enjoyable, *Who Goes First*, by Dr Lawrence Altman (University of California Press, 1998).

What is so extraordinary is how long it took the doctors to cotton on to the fact that food was at the heart of this disease. It shows that, when it comes to diet, doctors have never had much of a clue. In five years at medical school I would be surprised if I received as much as three hours' training in nutrition.

Most of us would agree that what we stuff in our faces has a profound effect on our health, but we're also confused about what's good and what's not because of all the conflicting advice. Governments spend time and money berating us for not eating 'better', then come out with guidelines which are based on the flimsiest of evidence, for example, eggs. Recommendations for 'safe' levels of egg consumption vary ten-fold depending on who you listen to. In Britain 'official' advice comes from the unfortunately named COMA – the Committee on Medical Aspects on Food Policy. They say stick to one egg a week. The World Health Organization (WHO) seem happy to recommend a safe limit of ten eggs a week. However, there is zero evidence that in a normal population egg consumption has *any* measurable impact on health or life expectancy. It's all part of the cholesterol mythology, something dealt with in detail later.

CAN WE BELIEVE ANYTHING?

Most people are justifiably sceptical about what they read and hear because much of the evidence appears to change from week to week. Although this is to some extent true, there are areas of research where the evidence has been steadily mounting year on year. Our relationship with food is complex, which explains why some of the conclusions coming out of modern studies appear paradoxical. For example:

- Eating fruit and vegetables dramatically lowers your risk of dying from cancer or heart disease

- But taking supplements of betacarotene, a chemical compound found in certain vegetables, increases your chances of dying from cancer and heart disease

- Heart disease is a common cause of death, and high levels of cholesterol in the blood are associated with heart disease

- Yet blood cholesterol levels are irrelevant as a predictor of who will die

- Men who drink moderate amounts of alcohol live longer than those who don't drink at all or those who drink a lot

- Research on rodents in the 1960s showed that nitrates are carcinogenic, yet people with high levels of nitrates in their diet are better protected against cancer than those exposed to low levels

All these statements have a large and consistent body of scientific evidence behind them. Some are surprising, some are not.

WHO'S TO BLAME?

'My opinions may have changed, but not the fact that I am right.'

Ashleigh Brilliant

Part of the reason for so much confusion is because of the unholy alliance of reporters, scientists, pressure groups and a food industry only too keen to put two and two together and make a million.

The media, of course, likes a good story. Newspapers and television reporters are paid to deliver fresh, surprising and highly exaggerated nuggets of news. Headlines I've enjoyed recently include: 'Town panics at killer disease in ostrich abattoir', 'Mutant virus ate my face' and 'Mad Cow Disease will kill 10 million, says scientist.'

Newspapers can even run completely contradictory stories one after the other quite happily. The same newspaper ran these headlines within days of each other: Vitamin E 'reduces risk of coronary' and Vitamin E pills 'may be harmful'.

Scientists are also to blame because they tend to leap on trends and thrash them to death. Although they like to think of themselves as impartial and unwilling to go beyond the facts, the ones I know are just as keen to make their name as the rest of us. They do a piece of research, then often draw quite unwarranted conclusions. The first, and most common trick, is what is known in the trade as the Ratamorphic fallacy.

You give a rat, mouse or some other unfortunate rodent substance X. The rodent develops cancer. Or perhaps the rodent is cured of a cancer that the scientist gave it in the first place. Either way you've got a headline and a research grant.

Unfortunately, what is now clear is that tests done on rodents are of very limited relevance to humans. Professor Bruce Ames of the University of California is a noted critic of the way that experiments in animals have been used to generate cancer scares. He argues, for example, that there is no evidence that our health is being undermined by pesticides. As he and others have pointed out, 99.99 per cent of the pesticides that we consume are natural, in the sense that they are produced by plants and vegetables to ward off and repel insect attack. Although critics have tried to draw a distinction between synthetic and natural pesticides, the reality is that, like synthetics, most natural pesticides will induce cancers in rats and mice. As Bruce Ames says, this does not mean they will do so in humans:

> Over a thousand chemicals have been reported in roasted coffee: only twenty-eight have so far been tested and more than half of those (nineteen) are rodent carcinogens. This does not mean that coffee is dangerous but rather that animal cancer tests and worst-case risk assessment build in enormous safety factors and should not be considered true risks.

On the basis of animal studies, researchers have put forward the theory that drinking coffee causes cancer of the colon. This theory has been tested and re-tested in human populations only to produce completely the opposite conclusions.

There is no doubt that in high doses some pesticides can be extremely toxic to people who are exposed to them, and dangerous to wildlife. Pesticides are a significant health risk for farmers and people who spray crops, but not for the general population who eat that food. Although the proposition seems reasonable, it simply isn't true that just because a chemical causes cell damage at very high doses it will cause damage at low doses.

There are many reasons for this. We humans are blessed with fabulous defence mechanisms, enzymes that can chew, break up and get rid of most of the chemicals, natural or synthetic, that are thrown at us. These defence mechanisms can, however, be swamped by very large doses of chemicals. Paracetamol is one example. Normally paracetamol is broken down into harmless constituents by enzymes in the body and then excreted in the urine. However, if you take a paracetamol overdose – say over twenty tablets in one go – then the normal enzyme system is overwhelmed. Instead of breaking the paracetamol down into something harmless, your body takes it down a different metabolic pathway. The result is a toxic chemical that can severely damage the liver. On the other hand, the danger is not cumulative – you can take a paracetamol every day of your life and it will not cause liver failure. The paradox is that paracetamol overdose is the leading cause of liver transplant in this country, yet paracetamol is also one of the safest, most widely used drugs in the world. The same principle applies to pesticides.

Nitrates are Good for You...

A clear example of how the Ratamorphic fallacy can lead you astray is found in nitrates. For decades it has been assumed that the nitrates we consume in our food and water are bad for our health and governments have tried to reduce their levels. The belief that nitrates are bad for you is based largely on research done thirty years ago in rodents. At the time it was found that a bi-product of nitrates could cause cancer in the rodents and ever since scientists have been hunting for evidence that it causes cancer in humans. What they have found is the opposite.

Professor David Foreman of the University of Leeds, and formerly of the Imperial Cancer Research Fund, has spent years studying the effects of nitrates in humans: 'What I and others have found is that the populations in the UK with the highest levels of stomach cancer, such as people in North Wales, have some of the lowest exposures to nitrates. In contrast, the population of East Anglia, which has some of the highest nitrate exposure levels, have relatively low levels of stomach cancer.'

His conclusion is that 'All the research that we've done on cancer of the stomach would not indicate a direct association with nitrate, either from drinking water or from food components.'

A study published in the *British Journal of Cancer* makes the same point. In this study, started in 1985, 120,000 Dutch men and women were observed for a period of years to see who would develop stomach cancer. Six years into the study 219 men and sixty-three women had done so. The study found that those ingesting the most nitrates in their food and drink were least likely to get stomach cancer. This finding has been consistently repeated in other studies and other countries.[1]

Far from being harmful, nitrates may even be a beneficial component of our diet. That's because nitrates do something in humans that studies in rodents had never suggested. But to tell the story properly I have to step back a stage and look at why we lick our wounds.

WHY LICKING WOUNDS IS GOOD FOR THEM

When you cut yourself your natural instinct is to lick the wound. We do it, dogs do it, even rats do it. Intrigued by this, Professor Nigel Benjamin of St Bartholomew's Hospital, London decided to investigate further.[2] What he and his colleagues found was then when you lick your hand the nitrates in your saliva, which come from your diet, react with your skin to produce an invisible but highly poisonous gas, nitric oxide. This gas is effective at killing the bacteria and micro-organisms that might otherwise cause an infection on the skin.

Licking wounds therefore is clearly a good idea. Professor Benjamin and his team looked further. In a series of gruesome self-experiments they fed tubes down their noses and into their stomachs. Then they ate lettuce, which is rich in nitrates, and collected the gas being generated in their stomachs. When they measured this they found that it contained very high levels of nitric oxide, levels which would rapidly kill most bacteria.

Further investigations involved schoolboys from Eton College trekking in Nepal and Tibet. Half the boys were given nitrate tablets, which they ate with their normal meals. The boys who ate the nitrate tablets had less diarrhoea and far fewer infections than the rest of the boys.

It turns out that nitric oxide is particularly good at killing some of the more dangerous pathogens to be found in our food: e-coli 0157, for example. A recent outbreak of this in Scotland killed more than twenty people – a world record. Our first line of defence against most of the dangerous bacteria we eat is stomach acid. But as Dr Roelf Dijkuizen of Aberdeeen University has discovered, e-coli 0157 is particularly resistant to acid. His experiments show that e-coli 0157 can survive for up to two hours when exposed to stomach acid alone. The presence of a small amount of nitric oxide, however, leads to complete and rapid destruction of the e-coli. As Dr Dijkuizen points out: 'It almost looks as if the scientific community is making a complete circle. First of all the research was done into how harmful nitrate could be by causing gastric cancer. Then it was found that there was no relationship and that nitrates don't cause gastric cancer. Now we're looking into how good it can be for you.'

The nitrate story is fascinating because it shows just how complicated the world really is. The Green movement is almost certainly right when they claim that nitrates from fertilizers washing into rivers are damaging to the environment and should be discouraged for those reasons. But as for being bad for our health? The case is not proven. What you can conclude from the research is that:

- There is no good evidence that nitrates cause cancer

- There is excellent evidence that eating vegetables protects against cancer

- Eating a bowl of lettuce before your meal, as the French and Americans do, will probably help your body kill any dangerous bacteria that may be hidden in your food

WHY ALCOHOL IS GOOD FOR YOU...

Alcohol is the most used and abused drug in the world. It brings enormous pleasure and enormous pain. Using the same logic as with pesticides, people have assumed that because large amounts of alcohol are very damaging, small amounts must be a bit damaging. This is not true.

Drinking too much alcohol can certainly lead to cirrhosis, cancer, vomit on your carpet and being run over by a bus. But in moderate amounts alcohol can be life-enhancing and confers a number of useful health benefits.

Studies were carried out as long ago as 1926 which showed that people who drank moderate amounts of alcohol lived longer than either those who drank a lot or those who didn't drink at all. This observation was totally ignored by the medical profession. In fact, the belief that alcohol is bad for you was so deeply ingrained that the idea that small amounts might be good for you has only really been taken seriously in the last ten years. A report published in the *BMJ* showed that the death rate in men was roughly the same for those drinking nothing or virtually nothing, and those drinking forty units a week.

The main way that alcohol extends life is by reducing heart disease. The evidence for this is now overwhelming. Its effect is so large that it cuts the risk of heart disease by at least half. Since heart disease is such a common cause of death it is not surprising that alcohol has a great effect on your chance of dying.[3] The link between alcohol and heart disease is probably strongest for wine, although the consensus amongst cardiologists now is that it is the alcohol rather than the type of drink which really matters.

How Does it Work?

Alcohol reduces the chance of a fatal heart attack in a number of different ways. There are essentially two stages to a heart attack. The first is the build-up of fatty plaque in the walls of the coronary arteries that supply blood to the muscle of the heart. The result is severe narrowing of these vessels which, though bad, is not fatal. A heart attack occurs when a travelling blood clot lodges in the narrowed coronary artery, abruptly cutting off the blood supply to that part of the heart muscle. It dies and so, sometimes, do you. Alcohol has beneficial effects on both these stages: it reduces build-up of the fatty plaque and reduces the chances of blood clots forming. This ability to reduce blood-clot formation helps explain some of the apparent paradoxes of alcohol. One of these is that while drinking a moderate amount frequently will halve your risk of a heart attack, drinking the same amount in one go will double it.

How Much and How Often?

Most cardiologists favour a few glasses of wine each night, and this is supported by the research. One study compared the lifestyle of 11,511 male and female Australians who had had heart attacks with 6,077 randomly selected fellow Australians from the same area who hadn't. What they found, after adjusting for age, smoking and medical history, is that for maximum heart protection men needed to be downing one to four units a day, and for women to be sinking one to two drinks daily.[4] A unit is a glass of wine, a tot of spirits, half a pint of beer. Doing that seemed to cut the risk of having a heart attack by well over half. More than nine drinks a day and the benefits disappeared. And binge drinking doubled your chance of a heart attack.

This ties in with the explanation that alcohol works primarily by reducing the formation of blood clots. As this is only a temporary effect, lasting less than twenty-four hours, you will be protected for the day following the drink, but not for the day after that. So drinking heavily on Saturday will not help build up your resistance for the rest of the week.

There is a final note of caution in this study and pretty well every study on the beneficial effects of alcohol, namely: 'caution is needed in promoting alcohol consumption because the adverse effects of abuse may well outweigh any potentially beneficial effect in reducing heart disease'.[5]

It is ironic that doctors are afraid of the good news getting out to the public, given that as a profession in terms of alcohol consumption we are seen to rank alongside travelling salesmen. Theories abound as to why this should be so, but it probably starts at medical school where one way to cope with humiliation and stress is to drink ten pints and drop your trousers. This behaviour is well tolerated and in some cases encouraged. One London teaching hospital used to boast a gentlemen's club which you could only join if your liver was palpable at the umbilicus (a normal liver fits neatly under the rib-cage on the right). My suspicion that doctors are proud of their coping mechanisms for stress is confirmed whenever I do an after-dinner speech: 'How many of you have phoned the BMA stress-line?' (silence) 'How many of you drink like fish?' (huge roar of recognition.)

An alternative theory as to why doctors drink was offered by broadcaster Pete McCarthy in *The Hangover Show*: 'It gives them something to do while they're smoking'.

Other Drawbacks?

There's a depressing list of side-effects that doctors reel off as a cheap and largely ineffective way to frighten people off alcohol: anxiety, depression, insomnia, dementia, gastritis, oesophagitis, cirrhosis, blackouts, fits, burning legs, chest pains, bronchitis, pneumonia, back ache, rheumatism, gout, obesity, infertility, acne and sweat rash to name just a few. Most of these are only relevant if you're a heavy drinker, but there is one side-effect in that list that's relevant even to moderate drinkers. It's number eighteen, infertility.

A recent study suggests that moderate alcohol consumption affects fertility, at least in women.[6] In the study 430 Danish couples trying to conceive were asked about their sex lives and personal habits. Sixty-four per cent of those consuming fewer than five drinks a week did so as compared with 55 per cent of those having more than five drinks a week. The more the women drank the less likely they were to conceive. The up-side of this story is that if you don't want to get pregnant then drinking is obviously for you. Since the effects are cleared from the system within twenty-four hours, if you want to get pregnant, just cut down drinking. Strangely enough, this does not seem to apply to male fertility. This study, and a number of others have suggested that moderate alcohol drinking has no measurable effect on the quality or availability of semen. This contradicts the advice infertile men are normally offered.

Hangovers

Finally, a brief digression about the evidence-based hangover remedy. There are a lot of remedies about, ranging from Pliny the Elder's favourite (fresh owl eggs) to prairie oysters and black coffee. Few have been properly tested.

Alcohol is absorbed into your blood stream from the stomach and small intestine. As alcohol is highly water soluble, if you line your stomach with fat before you start boozing this will slow down absorption and may help reduce the final hangover. Some people advocate drinking a pint of milk before going out on the town. When alcohol reaches your brain, it alters cell membranes and neuro-transmitter function. If this disruption reaches a certain critical level, you may find yourself singing songs like 'Get 'em Down, You Zulu Warriors' with your moleskins at your ankles. That's the fun bit.

What alcohol also does, however, is stimulate the part of the brain called the pituitary gland. This in turn stimulates water loss so that you end up losing more fluid through your bladder than you're putting in through your mouth. The more you drink, the more often you urinate and the more dehydrated you become. The water is drained from your whole body including your brain, which shrinks – and that hurts. A partial solution to hangover, therefore, is to drink plenty of water and take a couple of paracetamol just before you go to bed.[7]

But that is not the complete story, says Dr Ian Calder, an anaesthetist at London's National Hospital for Neurology and Neurosurgery who did a trawl of the literature. (Interestingly, anaesthetists have the highest rates of cirrhosis of the liver of any specialists in medicine.) The major component of alcohol is ethanol, but Dr Calder doesn't believe ethanol is the villain.

Ethanol itself may play only a minor part in producing the thirst, headache, fatigue, nausea, sweating, tremor, remorse and anxiety that hangover sufferers report. Hangover symptoms are worst at a time when almost all ethanol and its metabolite acetaldehyde have been cleared from the blood. Between a quarter and a half of drinkers claim not to experience hangover symptoms despite having been intoxicated.

He thinks that it is the methanol (as in meths), not the ethanol content of alcohol, that is to blame. Some drinks contain up to 2 per cent methanol, and these are also the drinks that research in volunteers show produce the most stonking hangovers.[8] Listed in order of that ability to produce hangovers they are: brandy, red wine, rum, whisky, white wine, gin, vodka, and pure ethanol.

The problem with methanol, apart from the fact that in large doses it makes you blind, is that your liver breaks it down into formic acid, which is vicious, poisonous stuff. You can slow the breakdown of methanol into formic acid by drinking more ethanol, so the idea of the 'hair of the dog' is based on solid biochemistry.

WHY COFFEE AND TEA DRINKERS GET LESS CANCER

As I mentioned earlier, there's some evidence that coffee, at least in huge quantities, causes cancer in rodents. A trawl through the research done on human beings, however, suggests that although there are theoretical reasons why it should cause colon cancer, there's little evidence that it actually does. In fact the reverse seems to be true. The *International Journal of Epidemiology* quotes: 'Attention has long been drawn to the potentially harmful effects of coffee on health, however recent epidemiological studies have suggested unexpected, possibly beneficial effects of coffee.'[9]

And there's more. *The European Journal of Cancer Prevention* found 'lower rates of colorectal cancer in tea and coffee drinkers'.[10]

Many studies on bowel cancer have found, almost incidentally, that coffee and tea are associated with a lower risk of these sort of cancers. For coffee there's no obvious explanation of why this should be the case, but amongst cancer researchers tea has certainly been a hot subject for some time. The tea story begins long ago in Japan where it was noticed that in one particular area the death rate from a number of cancers was much lower than in the rest of the country. The staple crop in that area is green tea which the locals slurp down every day. Excited by these findings, researchers went off to start experimenting on mice. One group of happy rodents drank extract of green tea all their lives while the others stuck to plain water. There was a big reduction in cancer deaths amongst the tea drinkers. This sparked worldwide tea research into both oriental green tea and our own black variety, much of it by Dr Mike Clifford of the University of Surrey, an expert in hot and cold beverages: 'We know from tissue studies that components of both green and black tea will inhibit the development of certain cancers which may be relevant to man. We also know from animal studies, particularly with reference to lung cancer and cancer of the oesophagus that both green and black tea could be protective.'

The average Britain drinks about three cups a day. As this includes those people who drink none, there must be many people who drink four or five cups a day. According to Mike Clifford, this: 'might well be enough to have an effect, I would have thought. We are currently investigating what effect adding milk might have, whether it helps or hinders, but we don't know the answer to that yet'.

We may not know the answer to the milk in tea debate but we do know why filter coffee is said to be better for you than unfiltered. According to the *BMJ* pouring boiling water onto ground coffee beans causes the release of dipterpenes, chemicals that react with your liver to increase blood cholesterol.[11] Drinking five mugs of coffee a day made this way would raise blood cholesterol levels by about 20 per cent. Filtering coffee removes dipterpenes and prevents this happening.

THE CHOLESTEROL DEBATE

How much does cholesterol really matter? For years the message has been simple: 'Cholesterol and fat will kill you, so eat less, you sad fat bastards.' I've sat behind my desk saying this sort of thing for years (couched perhaps in slightly kinder words) until I began to wonder whether all I was doing was just exercising my mouth. Health promotion of this type does not make a blind bit of difference. You don't have to take my word for it – that was the conclusion of a systematic review and analysis of randomized controlled trials in the *BMJ*: 'Counselling, education and drug treatments were ineffective in achieving reductions in total mortality or mortality from cardiovascular disease when used in general or workforce populations of middle-aged adults.'[12]

But why are we so obsessed by cholesterol? The short answer is that drug companies and food manufacturers have jumped on to the fat wagon and managed to persuade us that cholesterol is a word to be feared above all others. Cholesterol is a risk factor for heart disease, but nowhere near as important as most people think.

Pity the poor old Lithuanians. Life in the USSR was never great fun and since the break up of the Soviet Union it has in many ways become harder. It is perhaps not surprising that Lithuanian men have high rates of heart disease. In fact death rates from heart disease are four times higher in middle-aged Lithuanian men than in Swedish men of the same age.[13] Yet, as this study showed, the Lithuanian men had much higher rates of heart disease than the Swedes despite having *lower* blood cholesterol levels. Smoking rates were comparable between the two groups, but there was one other interesting difference I will come back to later.

Early attempts to treat high levels of blood cholesterol by drugs were effective in the sense that they reduced rates of heart disease in the men taking them; unfortunately the trials also showed that you were overall *more* likely to die if you were taking the drugs than if you weren't.

The latest generation of cholesterol-lowering drugs, the statins, do appear to reduce your risk of developing heart disease and dying. How impressed you are by the size of the effect depends largely on how the evidence is presented to you. But there is one oddity about cholesterol-lowering drugs and that is the fact that they appear to work just as effectively whatever cholesterol levels you start off with. As the *Journal of the American Medical Association* points out, this is not what should happen.[14] In fact, the *JAMA* article goes on to suggest that the protective effect of the drugs may have little to do with the drugs' cholesterol-lowering ability and more to do with their quite separate ability to reduce inflammation and the chances of clots forming.

Similarly, the world's largest and longest heart study has failed to find a significant link between deaths from heart attacks and high cholesterol levels. The Monica Study, which is sponsored by the World Health Organization (WHO) followed people in twenty-one different countries for over ten years. During that time over 150,000 of those being studied had heart attacks, mainly people in western Europe but also in Russia, Iceland, Canada, China and Australia. The good news, which came out in a preliminary report in 1998, was that rates of heart disease are dropping across Europe, Australia and North America. But this, apparently, had nothing to do with falling cholesterol levels because, well, they're not falling. Or, as the report puts it: 'Changing rates of coronary heart disease in different populations did not appear to relate at all well to the change in the standard risk factors.'

Inter-country comparisons are always difficult, because there are so many factors other than diet that affect people's lives. If you're living in a war zone, for example, then your cholesterol levels are likely to be a minor factor in your future health. So it is more convincing to take a group of men and women in one country, measure several different aspects, and follow them over time. This was done recently with a large group in Scotland.[15]

In this study, started in the early 1980s, researchers randomly selected 11,629 men and women aged 40 to 59, carried out their tests, then sat back to see who would die and of what. The results were surprising. 'Smoking, blood pressure and fibrinogen predicted coronary disease and also death, but other factors are less consistent.'

Although blood levels of cholesterol measured at the start of the study turned out to be a significant predictor of who would develop heart disease, they were an insignificant predictor of who would die. Smoking and a high blood pressure are well-known killers, but why is fibrinogen so important?

Clots

As I mentioned at the beginning of this chapter, alcohol reduces the chance of clots forming in your blood, lodging in blood vessels and causing a heart attack or stroke. The reason why increased levels of fibrinogen in your blood lead to death is that fibrinogen, which is naturally produced by your body, has the reverse effect, *increasing* the chance of clot formation.

Clots are now the subject of intense research and no doubt in a few years' time we'll see supermarket shelves bulging with foods saying 'clot free' or 'increases clotting times'. The drug companies are also interested in clotting, but they have a problem because a drug that is fabulously good at preventing clots forming is already on the market, and has been for over a hundred years – *aspirin*. Everyone who has heart disease or is a potential stroke victim should be on low-dose aspirin (75–150mg). One of the best things you can do for someone who has had a heart attack is to give them an aspirin immediately, as this will dramatically reduce their chance of dying. This is a difficult message to get across in the heat of the moment. A GP friend told me that recently one of his patients rang up to say her husband had just had what sounded like a heart attack. My friend told her to give him an aspirin while waiting for the ambulance. She was upset: 'My husband's dying and all you can say is take an aspirin. What sort of doctor are you?' and so on. She obviously felt his advice trivialized her husband's condition, but although it doesn't sound very impressive or high-tech, aspirin is one of the few pills that deserves the title 'miracle drug'.

For people who don't have heart disease, taking an aspirin a day is not a good idea as the side-effects, such as intestinal bleeding, outweigh the benefits. If you can't take aspirin but are keen to improve your clotting time you could try fish.

Fish

The diet of a nation not exactly renowned for its culinary flair has provided researchers with much food for thought. Eskimos chomp their way through mountains of blubber every year, and yet have low rates of heart disease. One reason is that they eat a lot of fish, and fish oils make your blood less likely to clot. This idea was tested a while back by a Cambridge professor who decided to try eating Eskimo-style for a hundred days.

For breakfast he had herring; for lunch, salmon; dinner, more salmon, shellfish and yet more salmon. For the truly authentic touch he imported and ate a seal. The diet was a success at first but he overdid it; the time his blood took to clot increased dramatically from four to fifty minutes, and he nearly died from internal bleeding.

The fish to eat are the oily ones, such as herring, mackerel or salmon. According to the *Journal of American Medical Association* eating fish cuts your risk of sudden cardiac death by about half. A study of 20,551 men aged 40 to 84 found those who ate fish once a week had a 52 per cent lower risk of sudden cardiac death – death within one hour of onset of symptoms – than those eating fish less than once a month.[16] Unfortunately, you don't get the same benefit from swallowing fish oil capsules.

Which Fats?

The message seems to have changed from 'fat is bad' to 'some fats are bad'. In essence, if it comes from an animal it's bad and from a vegetable or a fish it's good. Changing the type of fat you eat appears to be more effective than trying to cut down on fat, at least according to a study in the *New England Journal of Medicine*. Eighty thousand women aged between 34 and 59 years had their diets checked and were then followed for fourteen years. The principal finding should no longer be a big surprise, namely, total fat intake was not significantly related to the risk of coronary disease.[17]

What was discovered is that the type of fat the women ate was crucial. Switching from animal fats to olive oil and polyunsaturated margarines had a dramatic effect on the risk of heart disease. They estimated that 'the replacement of 5 per cent of energy from saturated fat with energy from unsaturated fats would reduce risk by 42 per cent'.

Seeing the effects on a large scale is particularly impressive. The Poles, like the Lithuanians, have for many years been the victims of rapidly rising rates of heart disease. Then, in 1991, this trend was impressively reversed.[18] Deaths for heart disease since 1991 have fallen by about a quarter. The scientists were puzzled: 'For most of the potentially explanatory variables considered, there were no corresponding changes in trend.'

In other words this dramatic change was *not* because the Poles suddenly started acting on top-quality health advice. They didn't stop smoking, didn't cut down their fat and they certainly didn't start guzzling lots of cholesterol-lowering drugs. Instead they did two quite simple things: they switched from eating animal fats to vegetable fats (consumption went up 48 per cent) and hugely increased the amount of fruit they imported and ate.

So, the message coming out of the research is that low-fat, low-cholesterol diets don't work because people don't stick to them and in any case they don't appear to reduce significantly the risk of heart disease. The diet to aim for is one high in fruit, vegetables, nuts and fish, the so-called Mediterranean diet. A recent trial from France on patients recovering from heart attacks was stopped early because the group on the Mediterranean diet were doing so much better than the control group.[19]

7|LIFE, DEATH & VITAMINS

Roughly two billion years ago micro-organisms first learnt how to use sunlight to convert water into food. Unfortunately this also produced an extremely toxic gas as a by-product. The gas was intensely corrosive and destroyed most living things, but the microbes didn't worry about that and just released it into the atmosphere. Over tens of millions of years the levels of this poison built and built, from virtually nothing to almost 21 per cent of the entire atmosphere. It was the worst outbreak of pollution that this world has ever known and led to the death of billions and billions of life forms. The gas that killed we now call oxygen.

What the micro-organisms had learnt to do was split water (H_2O) into oxygen and hydrogen. The hydrogen they mixed with carbon to make simple sugars i.e. food. They had no use for the oxygen, so they just released it. We think of oxygen as life giving, but it's actually very toxic. It reacts hungrily with proteins and enzymes, stopping them from working. It burns and destroys. If the levels of oxygen in our atmosphere rose much above what they are today trees would burst spontaneously into flames. The reason why oxygen levels haven't just gone on rising and rising is that eventually bacteria evolved an even smarter chemical trick – they learnt how to convert oxygen, the great poison, into energy. We, and all complex life forms, have inherited from them that ability. But it's a Faustian bargain, because although oxygen is essential to our life, it and its by-products are very damaging. There's now mounting agreement amongst researchers into ageing that oxygen-derived damage to cells is probably the main reason why we age and die.

A close analogy is a rusting car. You drive it out of the showroom in pristine condition; it is your baby, your one true love. But inevitably it gets bashed around, and as it does oxygen starts to do its evil work on the underlying metal. If you kept your car on Mars or Venus the odd dent wouldn't matter because no other planet has high levels of oxygen in its atmosphere. But back on earth it's an almost inevitable process; as iron is oxidized little rusty spots turn into big rusty spots. The car is ageing, it's falling apart.

In humans pretty much the same thing happens. We use oxygen to produce energy, but this process also generates a group of particularly vicious chemicals called free radicals. Once generated, these free radicals and other oxidants, such as hydrogen peroxide (the stuff that can turn you from a red-head into a peroxide blonde), surge around your body. They damage arteries and turn cholesterol rancid, which leads to the formation of fatty deposits in the arteries, then narrowing of the arteries, then heart attacks. It's that initial damage that starts everything else; if it wasn't for free radicals it wouldn't really matter what your cholesterol levels are – normal fat does not get deposited in healthy arteries. These oxidants also get into your cells and damage the DNA. If your body fails to repair this DNA damage the cell may become abnormal, and then cancerous. Cigarette smoking increases the level of circulating oxidants, and that's one way it causes heart disease and cancer.

Our cells make antioxidants in the form of enzymes which help suppress the build-up of dangerous free radicals, and there is some evidence that people who have naturally high levels of antioxidants live longer and have less disease. But there are other ways to boost your levels of antioxidants apart from having better genes, of which the most important is by eating fruit and vegetables.

FRUIT AND VEGETABLES

I wondered why fruit and vegetables are so good for you, so I asked a friendly biochemist. She said:

> 'It's because they are full of antioxidants'.
> 'But why do vegetables make antioxidants?'
> 'Because they make oxygen.'
> 'Oh, yeah.'

...which is obvious, when you think of it. Green plants use sunlight to convert carbon dioxide into food, and they breathe out oxygen. Since oxygen is such a toxic gas plants have had to evolve sophisticated ways of limiting the amount of damage that this oxygen does to them. Plants defend themselves against oxygen attack by sucking up selenium from the soil (it's a metal, but also an antioxidant) and by producing a wide range of different types of antioxidants such as vitamins A, C, E and betacarotene.

The evidence that eating fruit and vegetables is good for you is overwhelming. There have been literally dozens of international studies on the link between diet and chronic disease and these studies all say exactly the same thing (which is a rare, rare thing in science). For example, in one study, they followed 832 middle-aged men for 20 years to find out what the effects of eating fruit and vegetables had on their chance of having a stroke.[1] The men were divided into five groups depending on how much they were eating. The lowest group were eating less than 2 servings of fruit and vegetables a day and the highest group an impressive 8 to 19 servings a day. A serving was roughly half a cup of fruits or vegetables, 60ml of tomato sauce (strangely enough tomato sauce seems to contain more potent antioxidants than real tomatoes), 28g of chips, or a single potato.

The study showed that the more fruit and vegetables they ate, the less likely they were to have a stroke. Nineteen per cent of the men eating very little fruit had a stroke compared with only 8 per cent of men eating the highest amount.

If you're intrigued by the finding that tomato sauce helps prevent stroke, I refer you to the *American Journal of Epidemiology*.[2] This study of antioxidant status and heart attacks in European men showed that cooked and processed tomatoes have high levels of a carotenoid called lycopene. The findings were 'a surprise'. The lead researcher, Dr Lenore Kohlmeier, thinks we should be urging patients to add tomato sauce, ketchup, and similar products to their daily diet: 'We're not just giving the old advice about eating more fresh fruits and vegetables for a healthy heart. You will get some lycopene with a glass of tomato juice, and some is better than none. But for "high octane" lycopene, then go for the tomato products.'

Being a doctor, of course, he's also a killjoy and adds this rider: 'You're not going to prevent heart disease by eating pizza or chips with ketchup and counting on lycopene to save you.'

As I mentioned above, one of the most impressive drops ever seen in national rates of heart disease was recently in Poland, where really all they did as a nation was start eating more fruit and vegetables (including vegetable oil). Similarly, the apparently paradoxical finding that middle aged Lithuanian men have a rate of heart disease that is four times higher than Swedish men of the same age[3] *despite* having *lower* blood cholesterol levels can be explained by the fact that Lithuanian men eat less fresh fruit and vegetables than Swedish men and have lower levels of antioxidants in their blood.

The benefits of fruit and vegetables are not just confined to boring diseases like heart disease and cancer. Sperm counts, Alzheimer's, skin tone and asthma are just a few of the other areas where fruit and veg eaters benefit. For example, a study of 2,650 schoolchildren found that those who rarely ate fresh fruit had weaker lungs than those who ate fruit more than once a day. This was particularly noticeable in children who wheezed.[4] When you consider that oxygen and its derivatives attack every system in your body it is perhaps not surprising that antioxidants will in turn benefit every system.

The take home message of all this is that people who eat a relatively large quantity of fruit and vegetables (the recommended levels of five portions a day is way above what the average Briton eats) have a much lower risk of death and all sorts of diseases. It doesn't really matter if the food is fresh, frozen or tinned. Just don't boil it to death.

VITAMINS

Now, of course, having seen the wondrous effects fruit and vegetables have on health, it wasn't long before people started wondering how to jump on this particular wagon. If a carrot is good for you and carrots contain vitamins, let's extract the vitamins and throw away the boring old carrot. Unfortunately the world turns out to be a lot more complicated than that and carrots have had the last laugh.

For example, betacarotene – it was once the darling of both alternative practitioners and the medical world. Numerous studies had shown that carrots (an excellent natural source of betacarotene) have multiple good effects. So betacarotene was extracted and put in pill form and sold in numerous health food shops as the great cure all. But in 1996 there was a nasty shock for betacarotene guzzlers.

A large trial from Finland of 29,000 middle-aged smokers first suggested that suggested that taking betacarotene capsules actually *increased* your chance of dying from lung cancer and heart disease. Everyone was surprised and said, perhaps this is just a funny result. The hope was that other trials would produce different results. They didn't.

First up after the Finnish trial was the Physicians' Health Study.[5] This followed more than 22,000 American doctors treated with 50mg of betacarotene or placebo every other day for 12 years. They concluded that there was not the slightest measurable benefit to be found from taking betacarotene.

The results of another big study done by the US National Cancer Institute were even worse. The Beta-Carotene and Retinol Efficacy Trial

(CARET) studied more than 18,000 people at high risk of getting lung cancer because they were cigarette smokers or had been exposed to asbestos. They then either took betacarotene (30mg) or placebo and were followed for about four years. This trial had to be stopped early because they realized that one of the groups was dying much faster than the other. In fact it turned out that there was a whopping 28 per cent increase in deaths from cancer amongst the betacarotene consumers over the placebo takers.

Now, this was all clearly very puzzling and left the researchers scratching their collective heads. After further investigations they decided that carrots (and, by extension, other vegetables) are a lot more complex than just the odd antioxidant. They contain a rich mixture of micro nutrients which have been finely balanced by evolution over millions of years to produce something which so far defies our analysis. Swamping your system with high doses of betacarotene may prevent the absorption of other, more important micro nutrients and also discourage your own cells from producing antioxidants. I won't be rushing out to buy any.

SO WHAT SUPPLEMENTS, IF ANY, ARE WORTH TAKING?

Antioxidants come in every shape, size and colour, from vitamins to minerals. They are big business and if you pop down to your local health food shop you can quickly spend a large amount of money for very little benefit. I don't believe that the answer to every problem is to swallow more vitamins, but I also don't believe what I was taught at medical school, that as long as you have a decent diet you don't need to take anything else. This is clearly untrue – pregnant women are advised to take folic acid tablets to stop spina bifida occurring precisely because they won't get enough in their diet, however many sprouts they eat.

So, where do you start? Well you could either wade through huge piles of research papers which contain largely conflicting evidence or do what I did and phone up the world's leading free radical researchers to find out what supplements they themselves take...

Cathy Rice-Evans, Professor of Biochemistry at Guy's & St Thomas's Medical School, gave a typical response:

I take vitamin E and vitamin C. I take 300 milligrams of vitamin E every day and 250 milligrams of vitamin C. There is a considerable body of evidence to show that these particular antioxidants are protective against coronary heart disease and certain cancers.

> I already eat a healthy diet of natural antioxidants and other nutrients, but the levels that appear to offer protection are way above the sorts of levels we take in our regular diet. I think it's particularly advisable to supplement with vitamin E.

This would be music to the ears of Linus Pauling were he not dead. Linus Pauling is not as well known as Einstein or Crick and Watson, but he's certainly up there amongst the greats, one of the most original scientists of this century. He won two Nobel prizes in different fields and is seen as a founding father of modern biochemistry. He was doing very well for himself in the scientific arena until he published a book called *Vitamin C and the Common Cold* in 1970.

Pauling suggested that by taking incredibly high doses of vitamin C one could cut the number and severity of colds. This was heresy because everyone knew that the human body needs only a few micrograms of vitamin C; that's what we need to prevent scurvy, anything more is just waste. Yet here was Pauling suggesting that people take nearly 100 times that amount, or about a gram. It was clearly impossible to get that amount of vitamin C by sucking oranges and lemons, it could only be obtained by taking pills. The view amongst the medical profession then and now is that if you consume more vitamin C than you need your kidneys will just excrete it. So Pauling was, apparently, just producing expensive urine. Despite the jeers he went on taking huge amounts until he died aged 93, a good advertisement for his own ideas.

Well, Pauling was both right and wrong according to Professor Hemila of the Department of Public Health at the University of Helsinki in Finland, writing in the *Scandinavian Journal of Infectious Diseases*.

> Since 1971, twenty-one placebo-controlled studies have been made to establish whether vitamin C at a dosage of 1g or more a day affects the common cold. These studies have not found any consistent evidence that vitamin C supplementation reduces the incidence of the common cold in the general population. Nevertheless, in each of the twenty-one studies, vitamin C reduced the duration of episodes and the severity of the symptoms of the common cold by an average of 23 per cent.[6]

In other words it won't stop you getting a cold, but it may shorten the time you have it and make you feel better while you have it. He goes on to wonder why his fellow doctors are so convinced that vitamin C is a waste of money and concludes that it is because of a faulty review of the evidence written over 20 years ago by my hero Thomas Chalmers:

> For example, Chalmers did not consider the amount of vitamin C used in the studies and included in his meta-analysis was a study in which only 0.025–0.05g/day of vitamin C was administered to the test subjects. For some studies Chalmers used values that are inconsistent with the original published results. Using data from the same studies, we calculated that vitamin C (1–6g/day) decreased the duration of a cold by 21 per cent. The current notion that vitamin C has no effect on the common cold seems to be based in large part on a faulty review written two decades ago.

(I go into more detail on the common cold and what you can do to prevent or treat it in chapter 9.)

Is vitamin C good for anything else? Studies such as a recent one in the *BMJ* show that people with low levels of vitamin C in their blood are at much higher risk of heart disease.[7] The same is true of people who have had a stroke and people with lung cancer. However, none of this proves that taking vitamin C supplements will cut your risk of any of these conditions. The jury's still out.

If you don't want to wait for the jury to come back in and are contemplating consuming vitamin C pills on a regular basis it is probably wise to stick to the levels that Professor Rice Evans takes (250 mg) as there is some evidence that large doses of vitamin C can interfere with vitamin B_{12} absorption and metabolism. There is also evidence that people who are conditioned to eating high doses of vitamin C (over 1 g per day) develop a rebound reaction, which leads to lower than normal blood levels of ascorbic acid (vitamin C to you) when they stop. Theoretically you could then develop scurvy, which would be deeply ironic.

VITAMIN E

This is one of the best antioxidants in town and is the subject of intense research. A good reason to take vitamin E and C together is that they appear to be more effective that way than when taken separately (they potentiate). A lot of cardiologists I know take vitamin E, at least partly because you don't get that much of it in your diet. Principal sources are nuts, oil and whole grains. Frustratingly, the evidence for taking it, although quite compelling, is also confusing.

For example a study in the *Lancet* looked at 2,000 Finnish smokers who were given vitamin E (50mg/day), betacarotene (20mg/day) or placebo.[8] In this study the men didn't know what they were taking and were followed for five years. Of these men, 424 had 'major coronary events' over that period, i.e. either had a heart attack or died of a heart attack.

In essence, the study found that taking vitamin E did *not* cut your chances of having a fatal heart attack, but it *did* decrease your chance of a non-fatal heart attack (a risk reduction of 38 per cent). Oh, and by the way, in this study taking betacarotene increased your chances of having a fatal heart attack by about 75 per cent. Why vitamin E should be good at preventing non-fatal heart attacks and not much good at stopping you from dropping dead remains a bit of a mystery. It's possible that because they were taking quite low doses of vitamin E they didn't see the full effects.

The news is slightly clearer when it comes to cancer. Again it's Finnish men, this time 29,000 of them followed for eight years as part of a study by the US National Cancer Institute and the University of Helsinki, Finland. These men took either vitamin E or placebo. At the end of the study, there were 246 new cases of prostate cancer and sixty-two of them had died of the disease. Death rates were 41 per cent lower in the men taking vitamin E than in those who weren't.[9]

There's some evidence that vitamin E will slow the onset of Alzheimer's disease[10] and some evidence that it will enhance your immune system.[11] But don't overdo it. The maximum safe dose is about 800mg a day, considerably more than Professor Rice-Evans takes.

FOLIC ACID

Folic acid is an unfortunate name for a vitamin; although it's a member of the B group it has no number associated with it such as B_6. One suggestion I've heard is that it should be renamed B_4 as in the 'B_4-you-conceive pill'. The reason for the name change is that it's now widely accepted that taking folic acid before you become pregnant can stop most cases of spina bifida. What's less widely accepted is that folic acid may play a role in reducing heart disease.

Samantha is a young girl I met with spina bifida. Her spine failed to form properly in the womb and the lower half of her body is paralysed, leaving her with no control of her bladder or bowels. She'll never be able to walk and she has no feeling in her legs. Her mother Theresa is campaigning to try to stop tragedies like her daughter's happening again and again. 'She's had fractures of both knees, just from banging herself, and she's not even realized that she's broken her knee. When I look at Samantha sometimes and see how pretty she is and see some of the things I know she'd love to do I feel it is such a tragedy. It's all just so unnecessary.'

Each year in Britain over a thousand cases of spina bifida end up as late abortions. It occurs when the back of the developing embryo fails to close and the spinal cord is left exposed. The fact that tiny amounts of a cheap vitamin can prevent such a terrible birth defect from occurring is truly amazing. The risk of having a spina bifida child is at least halved if a woman takes 0.4mg of folic acid before she gets pregnant. This is one of the rare cases where eating vegetables is not going to do you as much good as taking it in pill form. The big and obvious problem is that most pregnancies are unplanned and taking folic acid when you know you are pregnant (at 6 to 8 weeks) is almost too late. It's something that the man who made the link between folic acid and spina bifida, Professor Nick Wald of St Bartholomew's Hospital, London, is passionate about: 'Many pregnancies, perhaps as many as a half, are unplanned, and if you're not expecting to have a baby you can't be expected to go out and get extra folic acid capsules. So what are we doing for the 50 per cent of pregnancies that are unplanned? We need some way of dealing with that. That's why some global or general public health strategy is needed such as fortification of a staple food with folic acid.'

Professor Wald and many other doctors are urging the British government to force millers to fortify our bread with extra folic acid. It's something the US government has recently done, and they've done it not just to prevent spina bifida, but because of the mounting evidence that folic acid helps keep our arteries healthy.

Folic acid does this by reducing the levels in the blood of a substance called homocysteine which, it is now thought, plays an important role in heart disease and strokes. No one I spoke to really knows how homocysteine raises the chances of heart attacks but it certainly does.[12] Professor Ian Graham did the research: 'We found that a high homocysteine level just about doubles the risk of having a heart attack or a stroke. We also found that the raised homocysteine level in the blood comes before the heart attack so it doesn't occur as a result of a heart attack.'

Earlier I mentioned the World Health Organization/Monica Study which compared heart disease rates between different countries across the world. I mentioned that none of the classic risk factors such as cholesterol were any good at predicting who would die of heart disease. Well, it turns out that homocysteine levels *are* strongly associated with who will die of cardiovascular disease (disease of the arteries, primarily heart disease and stroke).

In 1997 the *Lancet* published these figures based on data from the World Health Organization.[13] This showed that the Scots and Northern Irish share the honour of having the worst rates of heart disease and stroke in the world. They eat very little fruit and vegetables, so along with high levels of homocysteine they also have low levels of antioxidants in their blood.

More recent research has also suggested that giving patients with existing heart disease a mixture of folic acid and other vitamins may not only slow the thickening of the arteries but also reverse it.[14] It's all very suggestive, but the only way to find out is to do a proper trial giving some people at high risk of heart disease folic acid and others not. Such trials are underway.

VITAMIN B$_6$

B$_6$, also known as pyridoxine, is used by millions of women worldwide to treat the effects of pre-menstrual tension. Unfortunately I can't find any decent studies which suggest that it really helps pre-menstrual tension. Then again, not many decent studies have been done and the fact that it's taken by so many women clearly suggests it is, at the very least, an effective placebo.

In the UK there's been a lot of argument about B$_6$ because the government, on the advice of the Committee on Toxicity, has tried to limit sales of the vitamin to 10mg a day. It's done this on the dubious grounds that because very large doses can damage nerves, small doses may also be damaging.

As an editorial in the *Lancet* points out, this recommendation is based on some extraordinarily flimsy studies.[15] In one study researchers just talked to 172 women attending a private clinic and asked them if they remembered having any muscle weakness or numbness of the skin after taking B$_6$. This particular study has been widely savaged by the medical and scientific community.

Another study the committee quotes from involved injecting six dogs with huge doses of B$_6$, the human equivalent of 3g a day, about 300 times the 'safe' dose. The dogs developed nerve problems.

In the US the authorities have decided that it's safe to take ten times the proposed UK safe limit and the US National Academy of Sciences recently concluded that there's no real evidence of harm at doses of up to 200mg a day.

Clearly it would be a good idea if the people who are flogging B_6 for the treatment of pre-menstrual tension were prepared to fund proper trials to see if B_6 really does work, in the way that the cranberry juice manufacturers have for urinary tract infections. The danger for them is that they may get a result that they don't like. For the moment all you can really say about B_6 is, 'probably doesn't work, probably doesn't hurt'. Not a very catchy slogan and probably not the most persuasive sales pitch ever.

SELENIUM

Along with vitamins C and E, this antioxidant pops up quite regularly as a favourite supplement amongst free radical researchers. You mainly get it from fish, chicken, bread and cereals. In the *British Medical Journal* of all places there was a recent editorial urging us to take more.[16]

What worries the author, Dr Margaret Rayman, director for nutritional medicine at the University of Surrey, is that the amount of this essential trace element we are getting in our diet has fallen through the floor. 'In 1974, on average we ate 60 micrograms (mcg) a day, but recent figures show this has dropped to between 29 and 39mcg. In Britain, the official advice is that men should have 75mcg and women 60.'

Strangely enough this dramatic fall in the quality of British blood can reasonably be blamed on us joining the European Union. Before 1974 we used to import selenium-rich wheat from North America to make flour and bread. Now we use a lower-protein, lower-selenium European variety. That should give the anti-European element of the Conservative party something to shout about. The *BMJ* article goes on to point out why we should be all be worried about dropping blood levels of selenium:

Harmless viruses can become virulent by passing through a selenium-deficient host. This is an explanation for the first appearance of HIV in Zaire, a country with a selenium-deficient population, and for the appearance of new strains of influenza virus in China. A recent British study showed a significantly higher risk of spontaneous abortions in women with low concentrations of serum selenium. Sperm motility improved from 17.5 per cent to

35.1 per cent in subfertile men supplemented with selenium in a controlled double blind trial.

Dr Rayman is coordinator of the UK arm of an international study which will give selenium supplements of 200mcg a day to over 7,000 people and then see what happens. If you're worried about spontaneous abortion or want your sperm to be more motile, then supplements come in 100mcg or 200mcg. Don't take more than one a day. Or you could eat Brazil nuts, the richest natural source of selenium.

There are many, many other supplements around. Some may even be more effective than the ones I've listed above. Some, like DHEA (see below) are even at this moment being swallowed by professors of biochemistry somewhere on the planet. Time for me, however, to move on.

EXERCISE

For years now I've been urging my patients to do more exercise, then going home and slumping in front of the telly with a beer. I'm just not one of those people who believe 'no pain, no gain'. I neither pump weights nor jog, partly because most of the runners I know have knackered knees. I'm also not convinced that it makes much sense from an evolutionary perspective. It's hard to imagine that our distant ancestors, the hunter gatherers, did a lot of jogging or badminton. I see them more as gentle strollers, stopping to pick up the odd tasty morsel and only making a run for it when being chased by a leopard or a larger hunter-gatherer.

WALKING

If you want to develop big pecs and a flat stomach you're going to have to get down the gym and 'go for the burn', either that or have plastic surgery. But if you want to live a longer and healthier life, then walking is all you really need to do. I was surprised to find out just how much difference simple walking can make to your life expectancy. A study of male and female twins in Finland was particularly impressive.[17] Back in 1975 researchers collected together 8,000 male and 8,000 female twins aged 25 to 64. The twins answered lots of questions about their levels of physical activity. They were then divided into the following categories:

Couch potatoes – no real physical activity
Occasional exercisers – get out for a decent walk less than six times a month
Conditioning exercisers – people who did some vigorous walking or a spot of jogging for 30 minutes at least six times a month.

They followed these 16,000 twins for seventeen years, during which time 1,253 of them died, mainly of heart disease and cancer. Once they'd allowed for differences due to the amount people smoked and drank, death rates were calculated as 12 per cent for those who were sedentary, 7.4 per cent for occasional exercisers, and 4.9 per cent for conditioning exercisers. So doing the occasional bit of exercise cut their chance of dying by nearly a half.

Another study done in Honolulu came up with very similar results.[18] This time they took 707 retired men and asked them how much they walked each day. They then followed them for over 12 years. By then 208 of the men had died – 33 of heart disease, 19 from strokes, 68 from cancer and 88 from something else. The results were again unambiguous: the less you walked, the more likely you were to die.

The men who walked more than two miles a day had about half the chance of dropping dead over the ten-year period studied as the couch potatoes. Walking didn't just protect them against heart disease, but also cancer and other diseases. There is no form of medical intervention or pill taking that I know of that gets close to having such a big impact on our health as walking. Even a short walk to the shops seems to be better than nothing and, as I'll show in a later section on obesity, it's the only way to lose weight (but you knew that already, didn't you?).

SEX AND DEATH

Walking is, of course, not the only form of exercise. There is also sex. I love reading the Christmas issue of the *British Medical Journal* because that's when they let down their hair and publish some surprising and often witty studies. One of my favourites was 'Sex and Death: are they related?'[19]

Having an orgasm, at least in a man, is the energy equivalent of going for a leisurely stroll, but is it as healthy? Professor George Davey Smith and colleagues decided to check out the relationship between frequency of orgasm and mortality. As they point out, in many cultures male orgasms are seen as a bad thing, a waste of energy, depletion of the vital Yin: 'One of the extreme expressions of this idea is found among the

Huli people of Papua New Guinea. Here young men are sent to secret bachelor houses hidden in the forest and taught by celibate specialists of the mortal dangers of succumbing to women's desires.'

Chinese men are also keen on retaining their sperm. I remember a Chinese doctor telling me how he'd seen male patients who had made themselves infertile by attempting to hold on to their precious seed. The trick they learn is retrograde ejaculation; they somehow persuade their sperm to travel back up the urethra and into the bladder, rather than the normal route. It's not a trick that I'd encourage you to learn as it is apparently rather difficult to unlearn. A belief in the importance of holding on to the precious bodily fluid is also widespread in India. Mahatma Gandhi used to go to bed with young girls, not to have sex but to test his willpower. Again, Professor Smith has something to say on the subject: 'In North India any loss of semen is considered to be debilitating, leading to skin problems, lack of concentration, anxiety, painful joints, palpitations, headaches, pains in the chest, swollen gums and halitosis. The biological mechanism considered to be involved is that the production of one tablespoon of semen requires 40 kilograms of food.'

Anyway, Professor Smith and his colleagues decided to find out if there was any basis to these religious beliefs.

They chased up all the men in the town of Caerphilly, Wales, and five of the villages around it. The men all had to be between 45 and 59 when they started the study in 1979. The researchers took all the normal measurements of blood pressure, cholesterol etc. and then got stuck in with some detailed questionnaires, including the question of how often the men had sex. This is the great thing about being a researcher: you can ask the sort of question that would result in a punch in the mouth if you tried it out in the pub, and on the whole you get surprisingly honest answers. Most of the 1,222 men interviewed told all, and they were then grouped.

229 men fell into the 'High' category – twice a week or more
490 men were 'Medium' – less than twice a week, but more than once a month
190 were 'Low' – less than once a month.

The men who reported having the most sex tended to be non-manual workers and have slightly higher cholesterol levels than the once-a-monthers. Having collected together all this lovely information, the researchers sat back and waited to see who would die.

Over the following ten years 150 of the men died; 67 died from heart disease and 83 from other causes. What was found is that the more sex a man said he had per week, the less likely he was to die. The group having lots of sex, the highs, had half the risk of dying of the low sex group. They were not only having more fun, they were living longer. For men who are afraid that too much sex could be the death of them, this is clearly good news. The authors, in a slightly ironic tone, suggest that a campaign of 'more sex for a longer life' would be more effective than most other health promotion campaigns have been: 'Intervention programmes could also be considered, perhaps based on the exciting "At least five a day" campaign aimed at increasing fruit and vegetable consumption – although the number might have to be adjusted.'

One critic of this study pointed out that they hadn't really shown whether it was the orgasm or the sex that was providing the benefit. Is masturbation likely to prolong your life, rather than make you go blind and make your fingers drop off, as I was told at school? Good point. We clearly need a big study, something along the lines of 3,000 schoolboys followed for 25 years, half masturbating regularly, half abstaining. I look forward to reading the application grant. The critic also wanted to know if the men were married (they were) as studies have repeatedly shown that married people tend to live longer than unmarried people.[20]

What I wanted to know was whether women benefit as much as men from sex? A 25-year follow-up study suggests that, unlike men, it is not how often they do it but how much they enjoy it that affects a woman's life expectancy: 'This finding is compatible with a perception that the quantity of sexual activity is of more importance to men, while a greater concern with quality is seen among women.'[21]

The final word on this particular subject I leave with Professor Davey Smith, quoting from a study done in 1976 on 'Sexual life and frigidity among women developing acute myocardial infarction': 'Sexual dissatisfaction was found to be a risk factor for myocardial infarction with premature ejaculation and impotence in husbands being the major underlying factor.'

LIVING LONGER

So, is there anything that has been shown to actually prolong life significantly? The answer is 'yes', but you're not going to like it. Starvation, or, as its advocates like to say, 'undernutrition not malnutrition'.

For decades it has been known that if you keep a rat short of food from the moment of birth then that rat will live at least 30 per cent longer than normal rats, as well as being healthier as it ages. The rat must not be malnourished; it must receive a well-balanced diet, just a lot less than normal. The explanation of why this happens is back to the old enemy, oxygen. The cells in our body are continuously burning fuel to produce energy, and producing dangerous free radicals as an undesirable side-effect. The less efficient your body, the higher the metabolic rate, the more energy it has to burn to keep going, the more free radicals it produces. Free radicals, as we now know, are bad, bad, bad. One simple measure of your metabolic rate is your heart rate. If it's above 80 beats per minute when you're resting then its pretty high and you're pretty unfit.

In the animal kingdom there is a close correlation between metabolic rate and life span. Mice, who have high metabolic rates, rarely live beyond their fourth birthday. Turtles, on the other hand, with very slow metabolisms, can live for 70 years or more. There are exceptions. Birds, for example, live much longer than mice despite having high metabolic rates. That's because birds have much more efficient anti-oxidant mechanisms than mammals. Canaries, for example, have cells that are three times more resistant to oxidative damage than mammalian cells.

So how does starving help? Well, when you start to lose weight your body naturally slows down its metabolic rate to try and save energy (see the chapter on obesity). Studies on people who are fasting show that their metabolic rate is normal when they're moving around, but drops dramatically when they are resting or sleeping. So starvation leads to the consumption of less oxygen and the production of fewer free radicals.

Studies in monkeys also suggest that semi-starvation really does work. The National Institutes on Aging (a major research centre funded by the American government) have been doing what they euphemistically call 'calorie restriction' studies in rhesus monkeys since 1987. All the early signs are that calorie restriction is indeed slowing the rate at which the monkeys age. For example, calorie-restricted monkeys show a slower decline in DHEAS (dehydroepi-androsterone sulfate) and DHEA (the unsulfated form) levels than normal monkeys. DHEA and DHEAS are naturally occurring steroid hormones, hormones that your body stops producing as you get older. Dr Lane, who made this finding, says it's important but we mustn't read too much into it:

DHEA levels are of great interest to us, not because we believe that DHEA is the fountain of youth, but because it gives us a very good marker to measure rates of aging. It is important to distinguish between levels of DHEA that occur naturally in the body and decline with age and levels that are seen in people who pop DHEA pills to pharmacologically raise their natural levels in the hope of extending their lives. These artificially higher levels may not give them any benefit.

Many of the scientists who do this sort of research have put their stomachs on the line and are trying to keep their weight down to about two-thirds the level of what is regarded as normal to see what happens. I feel sorriest for the monkeys; they may have a long life but I doubt that it will be a particularly happy one.

Are you old for your age? Try this test to see how your body's responses compare to those of people of a similar age:

> Stand on your weaker leg. Close your eyes.
> Keep your planted foot still.
> How long can you stay like that before you fall over?
> If you're 20 you should be able to hold it for more than 30 seconds.
> If you're 40 you should be able to manage at least 15 seconds.
> If you're 60 then you'd do well to manage more than 5 seconds, so have a friend standing by.

If this test inspires you to seek further information, try contacting the following organizations: National Institutes on Aging at http://www.nih.gov/nia/ or Institute for Longevity Research at http://alpha.genebee.msu.su/.

8 | FROM SPERM TO BABY

CONTRACEPTION

The first proper guide to contraception and family planning was Marie Stopes's *Wise Parenthood* published in 1918. It caused outrage. The *News of the World* railed against it as a piece of filth (now that's ironic) and offered its readers who had over ten children a free tea tray. The funniest thing about the book is that Marie Stopes clearly didn't know her coitus interruptus from her coccyx. She advises her readers that the safest time to have sex is midway between the menstrual periods. If you don't know why that's hilarious then all will be revealed further on.

First though, a medical curiosity. Did you know it was possible to get pregnant by the oral route? A trawl of the medical literature finds this strange case from the *British Journal of Obstetrics and Gynaecology* under the sexy title 'Impregnation via the proximal gastrointestinal tract in a patient with an aplastic distal vagina'.[1]

A 15-year-old girl went to see her doctor complaining of cramps in her stomach. He discovered that she was nine months pregnant, but there was a bigger surprise. The girl had an abnormality of her vagina which made it physically impossible for her to be pregnant and yet she was. He did a caesarean section on her and delivered a healthy, bouncing boy. But how did it happen? According to the girl, nine months earlier she had been having oral sex with her boyfriend when a former lover popped up. He pulled out a knife and stabbed the girl in the stomach. She had an operation and the wound 'was explored…and the abdominal cavity washed out with sterile water'. No more was thought about it until the unfortunate girl discovered she was pregnant. What her doctor, Dr Douweouwe Verkuyl, now thinks happened is that she must have swallowed her boyfriend's sperm just before she was stabbed. The sperm leaked out of her stomach wound into the abdominal cavity, and from there were flushed to the fallopian tubes and made their own way into her womb. It sounds improbable, but it is published in a medical journal so it must be true.

METHODS OF CONTRACEPTION

Most of the time when people quote the reliability of different forms of contraception they are referring to the method rate, meaning this is what happens if you do it absolutely perfectly and by the book. Done that way almost any form of contraception is somewhere between 95 per cent and 99.99 per cent effective. But that's not what actually happens in the real world. If you're interested in real world failure rates, what's called the user rate, here are some drawn from the *American Journal of Public Health*.[2] These are annual failure rates for different contraceptive methods as used by members of the public in their everyday lives, as opposed to people in a study who are conscientiously trying to do the best they can. The figure on the right is the number of unplanned pregnancies that would occur in a single year if 100 women used that particular form of contraception.

	Failure Rate	
Trust to luck	85 per cent	85
Cervical cap	30 per cent	30
Sponge	30 per cent	30
Spermicides	21 per cent	21
Female condom	21 per cent	21
Occasional abstinence	21 per cent	21
Withdrawal	20 per cent	20
Diaphragm	18 per cent	18
Male condom	12 per cent	12
Progesterone-only pill	3 per cent	3
Hormonal IUD	0.60 per cent	0.6
Copper IUD	0.40 per cent	0.4
Injectable contraceptive	0.30 per cent	0.3
Sterilization-Tubal ligation	0.17 per cent	0.17
Combined oral contraceptive	0.08 per cent	0.08
Vasectomy	0.04 per cent	0.04

Looking at this list you can see why the female condom never took off. It also made me wonder what men are doing with their condoms that they have such a high failure rate. Perhaps they put them on afterwards.

IUDs (intra-uterine devices) are effective but have their own problems. They can lead to pain and heavy bleeding and they also increase the chances of getting a serious uterine infection (pelvic inflammatory disease), which may result in infertility. Having an IUD inside you also increases the chances of an ectopic pregnancy (the foetus implanting outside the womb). Although this is rare it can be extremely dangerous and often leads to emergency surgery. A recent study found an ectopic pregnancy rate of 0.02 per cent a year for women using a hormonal IUD, and 0.05 per cent a year for copper IUDs.[3]

There is Always the Morning After the Night Before...

A woman came rushing into my surgery recently urgently requesting 'the morning after' pill. 'How recently have you had sex?' I asked. 'About an hour ago.'

Although they call it the morning after pill, you're reasonably OK for up to seventy-two hours. I prescribed her a combined hormonal regimen, known as the Yuzpe method (the same hormones as you get in the pill, but at a much higher dose; they stop a fertilized egg implanting). It's the standard thing to do and it also turns out to be the wrong thing to do.

The World Health Organization carried out a study where they followed 2,000 women who had requested emergency contraception after a night of unprotected sex. The women either got the Yuzpe regimen (ethinyloestradiol 100µg plus levonorgestrel 500µg) or just levonorgestrel at a slightly higher dose (750µg). They found that when women were given levonorgestrel within 24 hours of unprotected sex, their chance of getting pregnant was 0.4 per cent; this was a lot better than the 2 per cent failure rate with the Yuzpe method. If they took it 49 to 72 hours after sex the failure rate of levonorgestrel rose to 2.7 per cent.[4]

The Oral Contraceptive Pill

My first experience of a real pill scare was back in 1995 when a number of newspapers ran as their headline story: 'Warning – using the new contraceptive pill doubles your chance of having a stroke and dying' with 'See your GP but don't panic' in tiny type further down the page.

The government's Committee on the Safety of Medicines (CSM), with all the sensitivity of a dead skunk, released the news to the media of a preliminary report which suggested that taking so-called 'third generation' oral contraceptive pills doubled a woman's risk of developing a thrombo-embolism. Their advice was that 'women should continue to take them only if they are intolerant of other oral contraceptives and prepared to accept the increased risk of thrombo-embolism.'

Soon I had a surgery with 200 worried women and two shopping bags full of returned Marvelon and Femodene. So I rang up the Medicines Control Agency (part of the CSM) and asked whether I could be sent copies of the three unpublished papers on which this advice was based. I was told, 'You are not allowed to see the evidence'. When I pointed out that this was for my personal analysis of the validity and reliability of the studies in question, the phone went dead. Thanks, guys. Predictably there was a huge surge in the abortion rate, with 2,700 extra abortions attributed to the pill scare in the first quarter of 1996 alone. Equally predictably, once the studies had been looked at properly there turned out to be no significant difference between third and second generation contraceptive pills in their tendency to produce clots.

Taking the pill, of whatever generation, will triple your chances of developing a clot in your veins. If you're on the pill for a year the risk of it happening goes up from 0.005 per cent to 0.015 per cent. The clots are inconvenient and painful, but only dangerous if they break off and bung up the lungs or cause a stroke. So what are your increased chances of dying? Well John Guillebaud, Professor of Family Planning at University College and Middlesex Hospital medical school, has done this calculation: 'If you take a million healthy women of child-bearing age who are not on the pill and follow them for a year, then fifty will develop a deep vein thrombosis and one will die of it. If you take a million women and put them on the pill and follow them for a year then 150 will develop a deep vein thrombosis and three will die of it.'

If you're on the pill you have an increased risk of dying of a thrombosis, up from one in a million to three in a million. Actually it is less than that because most of this increased risk is concentrated amongst women who smoke or have problems with high blood pressure. To put it in perspective, you are fifty times more likely to die in childbirth and about a thousand times more likely to die if you spend an hour scuba diving.[5]

Then in 1996 came my second pill scare, courtesy of the *Sunday Times*: 'Pill users face 10-year tumour risk'.

This was an odd headline because the study they were reporting on showed there was no added breast cancer risk at ten years. Presumably 'Pill users face *no* 10-year tumour risk' was not as dramatic. The basis of this headline was a study done by the Imperial Cancer Research Fund which pulled together research done on over 150,000 women from 54 different studies, and this was what they found:[6]

Increased risk of breast cancer	
Current pill users	24 per cent
1–4 years after stopping	16 per cent
5–9 years after stopping	7 per cent
10 years or more after stopping	Nil

The absolute risk of a current pill user getting breast cancer is small because it is a rare disease in young women. A guesstimate is that 300 out of the 25,000 new cases diagnosed each year are due to women being or having been on the pill. The *Lancet*, however, reported that the cancers found in women on the pill were *less* advanced than those in women who had never taken the pill. This is important, because it makes a huge difference to your chance of being cured if the cancer is caught before it gets out of the breast and into other parts of the body. So, on the one hand you have an increased chance of getting breast cancer on the pill, but on the other hand there's a decreased chance that it will be serious.

Apart from stopping you from becoming pregnant the pill does have other benefits. For starters it halves your chance of getting pelvic inflammatory disease, a major cause of infertility. It does this by thickening the cervical mucous, making it harder for bacteria to get into the womb. Since what the hormones are doing is putting you in a state that mimics pregnancy this makes sense from an evolutionary point of view.

Taking the pill also decreases your chance of getting endometrial cancer and halves your chance of getting ovarian cancer, a disease which in Britain kills 4,000 women a year. In this case the hormones make abnormal cells in the uterus commit suicide, 'apoptose' is the scientific term. I've still got those bags of Marvelon and Femodene. Any offers?

THE NATURAL ALTERNATIVES

There's an old joke that goes, 'What do you call people who practise the rhythm method?' Answer: 'Parents'. How we laughed.

A more up-to-date version of the joke might be, 'What do you call users of Personna, the self-styled *biggest thing to happen to contraception since the 1960s*?' The answer isn't funny. Well, not very.

The Personna contraceptive monitor was launched in a blaze of optimism in 1996. It's a modern way of doing natural family planning and is based on the fact that there are only a few days in any month when a woman can get pregnant. The danger days are detected by urinating onto a stick. Insert the stick into the machine, and, if it's a red light, no sex tonight. If used perfectly it's apparently 94 per cent effective, which still leaves 6 per cent of diligent users pregnant every year. Consider Rosemarie's story.

The reason Rosemarie went for Personna in the first place was because of the pill scare of 1995. When she read all the wonderful stuff in the papers about Personna she decided it was pretty well ideal. Down she went to her local chemist the first week that Personna came on the market. Every morning, along with tens of thousands of other women, she'd open the magic case and peer inside to see if the light for tonight was green or red.

When her periods stopped she wasn't worried. She had faith. But they didn't start again. Finally she decided she must be pregnant. She went back to chemist, where she had to pay for a pregnancy test, which must have been pretty galling. Being a gutsy lady she pointed out the irony to them and got a refund from them of the cost of the Personna kit (£49.95) which was better than nothing, but not likely to make a big financial contribution to the upkeep of the growing foetus. But it gets worse. Rosemarie went along for a thirteen-week scan and there on the screen were what looked like two heads. She's lying there thinking to herself, 'It's twins, it's twins, oh my god, it's twins,' when the midwife gives her the glad news that she's wrong – she's carrying triplets.

To be fair to the manufacturers, Personna has never tried to sell itself on its reliability, but rather on its naturalness. A method that is hormone free has its attractions, but after reading the literature I think I'd rather opt for the low-tech version of natural family planning. When used by motivated couples, taught by experienced teachers, the Family Planning Association says that natural family planning is 98 per cent effective. However, be warned that 'in the field' its failure rate ranges from 2 per cent to 20 per cent. To make it work properly you need a basic knowledge of female anatomy/physiology and ruthless self-discipline.

The Sympto-Thermal Method

This is the most effective form of natural family planning.

Most women have a twenty-eight-day cycle meaning that every twenty-eight days they ovulate, i.e. produce an egg. Unless it is fertilized by sperm the egg survives for less than twenty-four hours, so there is only one day in the whole month when a woman can get pregnant, when she has just ovulated. But there's a complication. Sperm can hang around for up to seven days inside a woman's womb waiting to ambush the egg, so if you've had sex up to a week before ovulating you are at risk of getting pregnant. Now the important bit – cervical secretions.

Before ovulation, a mucous plug blocks the sperm's route to the womb. As I mentioned earlier the plug is there to keep out any bacteria that may have swum up the vagina. But it's important that sperm get through, so, shortly before the egg emerges, the mucous plug becomes runny. The sperm can swim through just in time to meet the egg as it is released. Runny mucous is the sign that it's time to stop sex. What you learn at natural family planning classes is how to tell when your mucous is runny and when it's thick.

But that's not quite the end of the story, because you also need to know when you have ovulated so you can start having sex again. For that you need a thermometer beside the bed. Every morning you take your temperature (with a digital thermometer this takes sixty seconds) and chart it. When the egg is released, your temperature rises by a few tenths of a degree. This is the dangerous moment, the only twenty-four hours in the entire month when it is physically possible to become pregnant. A day or so later it's safe again.

The Calendar Method

Going by menstrual cycles is unreliable because most women's cycles are not completely regular. If you *want* to get pregnant, then ten to seventeen days after the beginning of your last period are the days when this is most likely to happen. These also happen to be the days (mid way between the menstrual cycles) that Marie Stopes advised her readers were the safest ones to have sex on.

If you're a red-haired, red-hot lover who wants it every night you're clearly going to have to compromise. Unless you're Catholic or allergic to latex there's no reason why you shouldn't mix your methods and use condoms during the danger period. A study in the *American Journal of Gynaecology* found this resulted in a failure rate of 2 per cent.[7] The majority of the failures were due to couples deciding, 'What the hell, let's risk it' and having unprotected sex at the wrong moment.

ADDITIONAL INFORMATION

The best source of information on the pros and cons of most forms of contraception is your local branch of the Family Planning Association.

You can find out about natural family planning courses through them or by contacting:

Fertility Awareness & Natural Family Planning Service UK
Clitherow House, 1 Blythe Mews
London W14 ONW
Tel 0171 371 1341
http://www.fertilityUK.org

MAKING BABIES

The advantage of knowing something about how your body works is that when you decide it's time to start making babies you'll know how to do it with maximum efficiency. She will, of course, start taking folic acid and he might think about dropping a few tabs of vitamin E and selenium (there is some evidence that both make for energetic sperm; see below). Apart from that there's not much more you can do to prepare yourself, unless you want to influence the sex of the child.

SEX SELECTION

Being able to select the sex of your future child has moved from being from being a theoretical potentiality to a practical, if rather complicated and expensive possibility. Forget all the business about douching with bicarbonate or standing on your head after having sex: none of these old wives tales appear to have any basis to them. They are at least less drastic than measures offered by 18th-century French travelling surgeons. These gentlemen would, apparently, offer aristocrats desperate for a male heir the option of having their left testicle cut off on the rather dubious grounds that boys only came from the right one.

These days we know, for example, that male sperm are smaller, faster and more abundant than female sperm and that slightly more boys are born than girls. We also know that more boys are born after wars, which is convenient because wars tend to result in the deaths of a lot of men, who then need replacing. Younger couples are also more likely to have boys. These two observations have spawned a theory that the more frequently you have sex in the build-up to conception the more likely you are to have a boy (soldiers returning from wars and young couples supposedly being more vigorous lovers).

The theories are great fun for academics to squabble over, but what in practice can help give you the child of your choice, and should couples have the right to choose anyway? I'm not against sex selection in principle, because if you've had four boys, I don't see why you shouldn't stack the odds in favour of a girl if you can. But it depends on how it's done. Getting pregnant, having a scan at twelve weeks and then aborting the foetus if it's the wrong sex is clearly the most straightforward way, but to most people that would be morally unacceptable.

A more complicated option is a variant on in vitro fertilization. In normal in vitro fertilization eggs and sperm are brought together in a dish ('dish babies' is a more accurate description than 'test-tube babies', but doesn't have quite the same ring). If it works, the resulting fertilized egg then starts to divide and divide again. When the embryos are sufficiently developed they are implanted. Thanks to a technique developed at the Hammersmith Hospital in London doctors can now take just one of those cells away from an eight-cell embryo and look at the chromosomes to check the sex. They can then implant embryos of the preferred sex. The fact that you can remove what is effectively a huge chunk of a growing embryo and it will still go on and develop into a normal human being is extraordinary.

In Britain sex selection is done using this technique, but is employed only to help people on medical grounds. For example, there are many couples who are at high risk of having a child with a genetic disease and some of these genetic diseases, such as haemophilia, affect only boys. So these couples are offered the option of choosing to have only girl embryos implanted. In Italy you can have the same thing done on purely social grounds, and I have certainly heard of couples who have gone over there to have it done. You'd have to be fairly desperate, because even in the best hands IVF is an uncertain business (in most centres the take-home baby rate hovers around 20 per cent, and in many centres it is far lower) and the drugs used to make the woman produce eggs have significant side-effects.

As an aside, it is very strange that in Italy, a Catholic country, doctors are allowed to do all sorts of things with embryos which are not permitted in Britain. Italy also has one of the lowest birth rates in the world, despite promulgations from the Pope against contraception. It's a weird world.

Ethically and medically the simplest form of sex selection would be one that involves separating out male and female sperm, then just squirting in the sex of your choice. The trouble is that people have tried this and not been spectacularly successful. The best known method is the so-called Ericson technique. The man's sperm sample is put through an albumen solution, a thickish fluid, the idea being that the smaller, faster swimming male sperm will find it easier to get through and gather at the bottom. Using this technique you could never hope to achieve 100 per cent success or anything like it. So what else is there?

Well, there is something that was developed in Cambridge, pioneered in cattle and which is now on offer to humans in Virginia, USA. The sperm are stained with a fluorescent dye which binds to DNA. Female sperm, being bigger, have more DNA in them than male sperm and glow more brightly when dyed. The sperm then pass through a machine that separates them on the basis of how much they glow. At the end of this process you're left with two little tubes, one containing boy sperm and one containing girl sperm. I've seen the machine in action up in Scotland and it is certainly very colourful, but is it safe having your sperm tie-dyed? I asked David Cran who's been pioneering its use in animals: 'Several hundred animals have been born after having had their sperm stained and been passed through the machine, and there have been absolutely no abnormalities.'

Which is not completely reassuring. The only way of telling how successful or dangerous it is is to try it out on humans, and that's going on in the United States at this moment. I'll pass.

INFERTILITY

If you haven't become pregnant after two years of trying then you probably have a problem that requires investigation. If the woman is over 35 you will have to react faster, a year being the maximum you can afford to wait before going for specialist help.

There are many reasons why couples might be infertile, but while doctors spend a lot of time investigating the woman it is just as likely that the problem lies with the man. Unfortunately there hasn't been a lot of decent research done on what, if anything, will help a man pep up his sperm. You should certainly give up smoking because that's an important cause of infertility and impotence, but after that you're down to the standard medical advice which consists of 'cut down on your drinking and wear boxer shorts'. The trouble is there is no evidence that either is particularly effective. As I mentioned earlier, unless you are an alcoholic there is little evidence that alcohol has any significant effect on sperm production. As for boxer shorts, well, it is important that the scrotum be kept cool, and boxer shorts are said to do this better than Y-fronts. But according to a study in the *British Journal of Urology* the Boxer Shorts Effect is a myth. In this study they took ninety-seven men who were being investigated for subfertility and measured the temperature of their scrotums. The average temperature of the scrotums of boxer short wearers was 33.8 degrees Celsius, while those wearing briefs actually weighed in at a slightly chillier 33.6 degrees C. The researchers also took sperm samples and found no difference in the quality or quantity of the sperm, whatever pants the men were wearing. Just to check they got them to swap underpants and re-measured. It made no difference.[8]

As I mentioned earlier, supplementing with vitamin E and selenium might help. In one study they persuaded nine men with low sperm counts to take vitamin E and selenium for six months. Over that period the men produced more normal and lively sperm than they had before taking the supplements, but unfortunately none of their partners became pregnant.[9] A study done in Glasgow giving sixty-nine men either placebo, selenium alone or selenium plus vitamins A, C and E was more successful. Five men (11 per cent) 'achieved paternity' in the supplementing groups compared to none in the placebo group.[10]

If you really want to worry about sperm and the future of the human race I recommend Debbie Cadbury's *The Feminisation of Nature* (Penguin, 1998). This book looks at the evidence that sperm counts have dropped drastically over the last fifty years and makes a compelling case for this one aspect of a much more worrying worldwide phenomenon affecting not only human beings but also animals ranging from fish to polar bears. The alarm bells really started ringing with a paper in 1992.[11] Danish researchers tracked down all the studies they could find from around the world on sperm counts and these added up to something truly alarming: it appeared that average sperm counts have fallen by *half* since the 1940s from 113 million per millimetre of ejaculate to a rather feeble 66 million per ml in 1990. You could reassure yourself with the thought, 'I may be only half the man my father was, but I'm making enough sperm every day to fertilize every woman in the UK and still have some left over for the rest of the world', which is theoretically true. The trouble is that in practice when sperm concentrations fall below about 20 million per ml, you get serious fertility problems. This study found that since the 1940s there had been a three-fold increase in the number of men dropping below the 20 million figure.

Further sperm counting studies have been done, with sometimes reassuring and sometimes worrying results. The Finns, for example, seem to have nothing to worry about in the trouser department, while the Scots certainly do. What now concerns a lot of scientists is that falling sperm levels may be part of a bigger picture which includes other disturbing trends such as a dramatic rise in testicular, prostate and breast cancer worldwide, and an increased tendency for alligators, fish and polar bears to change sex.

The best current theory that pulls all these phenomena together is that plastics, pesticides and other man-made substances contain chemicals that mimic the female hormone oestrogen. The fear is that by flooding the world with these products we have exposed ourselves and all other life forms to a chemical cocktail that may profoundly disrupt the balance of natural hormones. The future is becoming female and that's bad for all of us.

The scientists who work in this field don't have much in the way of practical suggestions as to how to reverse this trend or protect ourselves from it. You can try filtered water, but the process of filtering water through a plastic container and then through charcoal may actually leach out more chemicals than it removes. Spring water is uncontaminated at source, but it reaches us after a long exposure to a plastic bottle, and even if it were to come in a glass bottle, the glass might have been cleaned in detergents that contain chemicals that are oestrogenic.

Since these chemicals are mainly absorbed and concentrated in fat, not only our own but also that the animals we eat, the experts think that our best bet to reduce exposure is to cut down our consumption of animal fats. The research is at an early stage and there are plenty of critics, but what it does do is reinforce the argument that switching from eating dead animals and dairy products to something else is probably a good idea.

TESTING, TESTING

Assuming you do get pregnant, there are still many things that can go wrong, most of which won't and most of which are covered by any standard book on pregnancy. There are, however, a couple of areas where both standard books and your doctor are likely to offer you false reassurance. One is amniocentesis, which I've written about earlier, and the other is itching in pregnancy.

Many women itch during pregnancy, but really severe itching, particularly on the soles of the feet, or the palms of the hands, can be a warning that something is going wrong with the mother's liver. The condition is known as obstetric cholestasis (OC) and is quite common, affecting about one in every two hundred pregnancies. It is important to recognize and do something about OC because it can kill babies and make their mothers very sick. When I was at medical school we were taught that severe itching was common in pregnancy, nothing to worry about, and that women should be given anti-itch lotions, reassured and sent away. This is what happened to Jenny Chalmers. 'I had "take your nails and rake them down your body itching". I'd stick my hands in the freezer for as long as I could possibly bear them to be in the freezer, just to try and cool them because it just felt as if inside I was on fire.'

Her consultant said it was fine, nothing to worry about, it was normal. Then, when she was thirty-seven weeks pregnant, she noticed that the baby had stopped moving. Jenny was admitted to hospital. 'They brought in a scanner to look at the baby and then they just said, "We're really sorry, you know, it looks bad." They never actually said that the baby had died.'

Jenny's baby had died and no one could tell her why. Three years later, she became pregnant again and the itching returned, with a vengeance. Jenny begged them to do something about it, perhaps deliver the baby early, but the hospital staff decided this was unnecessary. At thirty-eight weeks she went into labour and was rushed to hospital. The doctors listened for a heartbeat and couldn't find one.

> The worst thing about stillbirth is that right up until the point of delivery, when you're pushing and pushing, there's a lot of noise, there's people encouraging you, the midwife's saying, 'Come on, Jen, push, push', and there's a lot of noise going on and then the baby comes out and it's just silence and you actually realize you are still waiting for that miracle, still waiting for that baby, your baby, to cry, and of course they don't. And I can remember saying to the midwife, 'It's another girl, isn't it?' and she said, 'Yes' and I fell apart.

It is now believed that undiagnosed obstetric cholestasis could be to blame for up to 20 per cent of late stillbirths and that is a tragedy because if the right diagnosis is made there is every chance that babies can be saved. So, if you have severe itching in late pregnancy, particularly on your hands and feet, ask your doctor for a liver function test. It's a simple blood test and could make all the difference.

FURTHER INFORMATION

A free booklet about obstetric cholestasis can got by sending an SAE to:

> The British Liver Trust
> P O Box 900
> Ipswich
> IP3 9QW

Jenny Chalmers runs a support service; for more information send a large SAE to:

> Obstetric Cholestasis Information and Support Service
> 4 Shenstone Close, Four Oaks
> Sutton Coldfield, Birmingham B74 4XB

BIRTH

My first introduction to the simple joys of birth was in 1985 when a kindly professor gathered his medical students round and promised us that the day we delivered our first baby would be the day we realized how wonderful medicine could be. When my turn came, I was allocated a twenty-year-old woman who shouted, 'Fucking hell, it hurts!' for about three days. When the baby finally arrived, it came out with the umbilical cord wrapped round the neck. I was on my own because the midwife had nipped out for a fag, so I grabbed a couple of clamps, stuck them on the cord, cut it, hiked out the baby and plonked it on the mother's stomach. Ten minutes of self-congratulation later, I reviewed my handiwork and realized that as well as clamping the cord, I had clamped two huge great tufts of pubic hair. I couldn't unclamp them without freeing the cord to bleed everywhere, so I opted for the scissors. This was not, I'm afraid, entirely successful and left a curious ripple effect. It is at times like these that you wish you carried a comb.

This was one of the few relatively normal deliveries that I have taken part in. That may seem strange coming from someone who has worked for six months on a labour ward, but the trouble with obstetrics is that you are only invited to the deliveries that go wrong. The midwives see all the joyous normal births and get all the chocolates, but if the baby becomes stuck or the mother explodes, then it's, 'Over to you, doc'. This is unfortunate because it tends to colour the doctor's view of what is normal and what is safe.

Like 98 per cent of couples, when our time came my wife (who is also a doctor) opted for a hospital birth for both our children, just to be safe. Every doctor I know seems to believe that hospitals are the only safe places for women in labour to be, but, is it true? A recent publication from the well-respected NHS Centre for Reviews and Dissemination, *Where Will You Have Your Baby, in Hospital or Home?* concluded: 'There's no evidence that hospital births are safer for all women and all babies, as long as there are no serious complications during pregnancy.'

A report from the Oxford National Perinatal Epidemiology Unit goes further: 'For some women it is possible but not proven that the iatrogenic risks associated with institutional delivery may be greater than any benefit conferred.'[12]

Iatrogenic means caused by medicine; they are saying that being in a medical setting attended by medics has risks that may outweigh the benefits. More of that later.

Where there are likely to be serious complications you're clearly better off in hospital. For example, if you're going to have a breach birth (when the baby's bottom tries to come out first) or have twins then the risks of the baby dying in a home birth delivery are large, about one in fourteen and one in seven respectively.

Now it is these sort of statistics, even when they don't apply to you, that frighten soon-to-be mothers. Alison is a low-risk pregnancy; she is under thirty, she does not have twins, the baby is head down, she has no medical problems such as diabetes or hypertension. Yet Alison is still terrified that something could go wrong:

> What if I need an emergency caesarean? I like the idea that if there are any complications I can be strapped to a foetal monitor, I'm hearing the baby's heart beat, everything is fine and the doctor is at hand, and the midwife at hand in the hospital nods and says, 'OK, it's all right,' that's going to be comforting to me.

Alison may find the idea of being surrounded by technology reassuring, but trials have found little significant benefit from the routine use of continuous electronic monitoring for low-risk women. What continuous foetal monitoring can and does do is lead to further interventions, as Donald Gibb, Consultant Obstetrician at King's College Hospital, London, concedes:

> That technology has certainly led to an increase in caesarean sections. This may have been due to failure of understanding of the technique during its introduction but in every hospital where you start doing electronic foetal monitoring, not having done it, you immediately put up the caesarean section rate.

Electronic foetal monitoring is not the same as putting your ear to the tummy and having a listen. It involves graphs and print-outs which the staff are rarely properly trained in interpreting. I remember as a junior doctor staring at the read-out which shows the baby's heart rate, and then it started to dip. This can be entirely normal, but everyone began to worry; the pressure was on to do something. Fear of litigation was nibbling away at the back of all our minds. A caesarean seemed like a good idea, and so it was done.

In the past thirty years the caesarean section rate in the UK has risen from less than 5 per cent to 17 per cent of all births. Nobody thinks this is a desperately good idea, but nobody quite knows who to blame. Is it scalpel happy docs, fear of litigation, or women wanting to 'keep their vaginas honeymoon sweet', as one notorious American ad puts it? On the surface it seems safest to blame the docs; after all what woman would opt to have herself cut open and then spend six weeks waiting for the wound to heal, while wrestling with a newborn infant?

Well, apparently many female doctors would, particularly female obstetricians. Armed with all the facts about the pros and cons of having a caesarean section versus a normal vaginal delivery, 31 per cent of London female obstetricians say that they would opt for the caesarean.[13] Of the ones who wanted a caesarean, 80 per cent said they did so because of the fear of possible perineal damage; they were afraid that the baby's head coming through would either rip the area around the vagina/anus or result in the appearance of a colleague with scissors who would do the same thing in a more controlled way (an episiotomy). Childbirth notoriously increases not only the risk of perineal damage but also the risk of damage to the muscles of the pelvic floor, which in turn increases the chances of becoming incontinent. Pelvic floor exercises are a great way of preventing this, but they are rarely done properly. Don't clench your buttocks or try straining as though you're giving birth; it's not about pushing or clenching. To find out which muscles I'm talking about try stopping yourself from urinating when you're in mid flow – it's them.

I have friends who have had caesareans who think they are wonderful, and others who felt it was a disaster, a failure on their part to have a proper birth. You can't condemn all caesarean sections out of hand because some are vital; as always it is the marginal ones that you wonder about. In broad terms the risks to a baby are greater from a vaginal delivery (though we are talking very small risks in most cases), while a planned caesarean section is probably two to three times more risky in terms of a life-threatening procedure to the mother than a normal birth. In addition, there are well-recognized complications to caesareans such as adhesions, intestinal obstruction, bladder injury, and rupture of the uterus next time you become pregnant.

Another friend of mine, Susan, recently went into hospital to have her baby. The little boy, Joe, was born and then suddenly became very ill. He was pale, sweaty, collapsed. The paediatricians rushed him to intensive care, where they found he had a serious infection. They resuscitated him, hooked him up to all the drips, poured in the antibiotics and after an agonizing wait, Joe started to respond. His parents are grateful to the hospital because they feel that without the immediate attention that Joe received he would have died. Susan now passionately believes that having a baby in hospital is the safest thing to do. What she does not accept is that Joe may have become ill simply because he was in hospital. About 14 per cent of people who go into hospital pick up an infection there that they did not have when they went in. Hospitals are unhealthy places.

I wouldn't like you to be left with the impression that I'm a whole- hearted convert to the joys of home birth, just that I think women have been oversold the benefits of hospital and undersold the advantages of being at home. I personally have done all the home deliveries I ever want to do. One in particular sticks in my mind. It was a water birth – Vivaldi wafting through the speakers, dad squatting behind mum buck-naked and the entire extended family (labrador included) squishing about in the foam. For all the encouragement, these affairs tend to take the best part of a weekend and, come Sunday night, the midwife was getting a tad bolshy: 'Push through your bottom, dear – like you're doing a number two!!!' I've never met a midwife who doesn't say this, and it has always struck me as tempting fate. Sure enough, out popped the mother of all number two's. Mum asked, 'Is it a boy or a girl?' and Dad chipped in with, 'How much does he weigh?' I almost popped it on the scales out of curiosity.

PAIN RELIEF

The main advantage of having children in hospital is pain relief. The first analgesic on offer is usually Entonox, a mixture of nitrous oxide and oxygen, which deadens the pain rather than removes it. It can also make you light-headed, liable to tears, laughter and the utterance of foul expletives which must never be repeated outside the labour ward.

The best pain reliever is the epidural, an anaesthetic injected into the spinal canal. My top tip is to book this in the car park on the way in because otherwise the midwife is sure to say, 'It's just coming out, no need to call the doctor now.' Three hours of sweating, swearing and screaming later they are still saying the same thing. If your hospital does them, ask for a walking epidural. It blocks the pain without blocking your ability to walk around, which in turn can help labour progress normally. It would also be good to know if the person doing the epidural has done many of them before.

I may never have been pregnant but I have had the experience of someone junior sticking a needle in my spine and I did not enjoy it. I had been vomiting like that nice woman in *The Exorcist* for three days and as for the headache – well, I've never known pain like it, doctor. I was sent to my local hospital, to see a consultant neurologist. 'I can't find anything much on examination, but we ought to do a CT scan and a lumbar puncture.' That's what I love about neurologists. None of this 'What are your concerns?/You must be very worried/Would you like me to hug you?' – just crisp, courteous, clinical efficiency.

The CT scanner showed a larger than average brain without any tumour but packed full of fresh and amusing insights into medicine. (Note: This is a joke. CT scans are very clever but they can't spot insights. You need an MRI scan for those.) As for the lumbar puncture, well, I was not looking forward to a needle in the spine but the registrar had seemed competent when I had met him a few hours earlier. Imagine my surprise when his junior trotted round the corner. Not just any junior, but one I had taught communication skills to as a student just two years ago. 'What are you like with pain?' said George. At this point I should have said, get me someone else, but the trouble is that, in those situations, you don't.

'I'm going to use a yellow needle,' said George. 'Great,' said I (yellow equals small). 'I'm colour blind though, so I have to be careful.'

George gives a great anaesthetic, which was just as well as it took him three goes do the lumbar puncture. 'I'm in slightly the wrong place here.' At last George was in and my spinal fluid was dripping out into bottles. He labelled them, filled in the forms and took them all the way down to the labs to get them done pronto. Unfortunately, he left his bleep by the bed and after it had gone off for the sixth time I felt obliged to answer it. The voice on the other end sounded senior. 'Is that George?' 'George isn't here.' 'Where is he?' 'He's gone to the labs.' 'Who are you?' 'I'm a patient. Who are you?' Cue dead phone.

There are other forms of pain relief available apart from an epidural, but they are rarely as effective. Some hospitals may still be using pethidine, but there is little evidence it works on the sort of pain associated with childbirth and a lot of evidence that it can affect the baby.

The main concern some people have over epidurals is that they may cause long-term back ache. A study done some time ago suggested that mothers who had had epidurals were more likely to have long-term back problems.[14] The problem with this study was that it was retrospective; they asked the women if they had had back ache before delivery and whether it had worsened after delivery. The women said no, they did not have it before, and yes, they did have it afterwards. QED. But later studies which have actually followed women before and after birth have found something quite different.[15] A lot of women have back ache before the birth, and that back ache just continues after the birth. In the retrospective study there seems to have been selective amnesia; the women had forgotten how bad their backs were before and then blamed the epidural for the back ache they had afterwards. There *is* an increased risk of back ache on the day after birth if you have had an epidural, but that passes with time.

INTERVENTIONS

Once upon a time (well, about thirty years ago) there was a list of 141 different forms of medical intervention that were considered essential for a birth to have a happy outcome. Women of a certain age will remember being given enemas and having all their pubic hair shaved off 'to cut down the risk of infection'. That list has been dramatically whittled down as most of these interventions have been shown to be useless. There is, however, one 'intervention' that studies have consistently shown really does help a normal labour come to a successful conclusion. Never mind the drip, never mind the doctor, never mind the midwife, never mind the pain relief, never mind anything else: the thing that will make a significant difference to labour is a companion, a companion the mother trusts, whom she knows and wants to have with her.

AFTER THE BIRTH

It is not the sort of thing that people want to talk about, but being depressed following the birth of a child is so common it is almost 'normal'. It's not what you expect because this is supposed to be a supremely happy moment, but it certainly occurs in over half of first time births. It's not just tiredness and stress, it's also because your oestrogen and progesterone levels go completely haywire. Most mothers recover by themselves, but in about 10 per cent of cases they don't. Their problem becomes chronic and this starts to affect the family and the child. One way of measuring if you're depressed is called the Edinburgh Postnatal Depression Scale, which is often administered by health visitors. You have to answer questions like:

> Have you stopped looking forward to the future with pleasure?
> Are you having difficulty sleeping because of anxiety?
> Have you thought about injuring yourself?

If you are tearful and feeling inexplicably negative about life then it's worth looking for help because if you are genuinely depressed you may not recover on your own. The trouble is that GPs are notoriously poor at detecting and treating depression (see later), whether it's post-natal or otherwise. This is surprising because so many seem depressed themselves. A few years ago I ran a communication course for GPs using simulated consultations. One of the scenarios was a depressed GP who had finally sought help after trying to treat himself. In the discussion that followed, it transpired that all the GPs in one of the small groups had been, or were currently, self-medicating with Prozac.

The research shows that if you fall outside the stereotype of what your GP expects a depressed person to look like (middle aged, unemployed, white, recently bereaved or separated) then they are unlikely to detect that you are depressed. In medicine we call it the Law of Halves:

- Half of people who suffer from depression go to their GPs
- Half of those who go are correctly diagnosed
- Half of those who are correctly diagnosed are correctly treated

This suggests that about an eighth of the people who need help get it, a figure which may be over-optimistic. One study looked at just over a hundred young mothers who had recently been seen by some sort of health professional (GP, health visitor, etc.). Three had been diagnosed as depressed and sent for specialist help. A review of these cases showed that the three who had been referred for help were not actually depressed, while the health professionals had managed to miss thirteen women in the group who really were depressed.[16]

To be fair it is a hard diagnosis to make because people will often deny being depressed because of fear of what others will think. I know a junior doctor who I will call 'Jane' who believes that if she admits to post-natal depression it will get back to her consultant and ruin her career. The trouble is, she may be right. Mental illness is a particular problem for doctors who, in the macho culture they have been brought up in, feel that they should be immune to such frailty. Since a diagnosis of depression can spell disaster for career prospects many go for months denying the problem and masking symptoms behind their professionalism. Jane is treating herself secretly with antidepressants and is terrified that she will be found out.

Another reason why many women don't go to the doctor is because they know they will probably just be offered drugs and they fear, quite wrongly, that the drugs are addictive. What you may not be told is that there are alternatives and the alternatives are as good if not better than the drugs. They are certainly better than doing nothing. A study in the *BMJ* looked at the treatments available.[17]

Over a nine-month period they asked women who gave birth in two Manchester hospitals to take the Edinburgh Postnatal Depression Test. From this they found 188 women who were seriously depressed. Despite being desperately unhappy, only half of them agreed to take part in the trial. The ones who refused to take part did so because they didn't want to be prescribed drugs.

The women were then randomly allocated to placebo, fluoxetine (an antidepressant better known as Prozac) or cognitive behavioural therapy. They found that the women who received treatment did much better than those who just got placebo, and that cognitive behavioural therapy was as effective as the drugs. More about drugs versus cognitive behavioural therapy and who you can get it from in the next chapter, where we discuss depression.

FURTHER INFORMATION:

More information about choice in childbirth is contained in *How to Get the Best from Maternity Services* available free of charge from the Department of Health, PO Box 410, Wetherby, LS23 7LN.

Information about local maternity services and support groups is available from Health Information First, freephone 0800 665544.

Information about home birth is contained in the leaflet *Where Should I Have My Baby?* Send an SAE to the National Childbirth Trust, Alexandra House, Oldham Terrace, London W3 6NH, or by telephoning 0181 992 8637. The National Childbirth Trust is a charity offering information and support during pregnancy, childbirth and early parenthood.

The Association for Improvements in Maternity Services – AIMS – offers information and advice on all aspects of maternity care, including parents' rights, technological interventions, natural childbirth and complaints procedures. A free copy of the AIMS publications list is available from AIMS Publications List, 2 Bacon Lane, Hayling Island, Hants PO11 0DN. Also available: *Antenatal Testing* – £3.00. Please include a large SAE. For general enquiries call 0181 960 5585.

9 COMMON, COMMON, COMMON

BACK ACHE

One of the consequences of our descent from the trees and attempts to walk upright has been back ache. At least 7 per cent of the adult population in Britain go to see their GP every year complaining about their backs. Most of them get a bit of advice, go away, and are never seen again. The doctors assume they're cured, and the textbooks are able to reassuringly assert that '80 to 90 per cent of attacks of low back pain recover in about six weeks, irrespective of the administration or type of treatment.'

But does the fact that patients don't come back really mean that they are cured or just that they have recognized that doctors can't do much about backs and have decided to go somewhere else? A paper in the *BMJ* set out to find out.[1] As the researchers point out: 'By the age of thirty years almost half the population will have experienced a substantive episode of low back pain. These figures simply do not fit with claims that 90 per cent of episodes of low back pain end in complete recovery.'

They chased up 490 patients who had gone to their GPs complaining of bad backs to see what had really become of them. Their conclusion was that 'Only 25 per cent of the patients who consulted about low back pain had fully recovered 12 months later.'

In other words the majority of patients with bad backs had just crawled away somewhere to endure their pain in a stoical British sort of way. This is unfortunate as there is now a lot of evidence that early intervention can prevent an acute problem turning you into a permanent back cripple.

Doctors are not very good at backs but it has not stopped us offering advice and treatment, some of which has been distinctly unhelpful, as Gordon Waddell, Professor of Orthopaedic Surgery in Glasgow acknowledges: 'The standard medical approach to back pain for the last 50 years or so has been to say, "Go to bed, rest...". All the evidence we have now is that that actually makes the disability worse.'

Professor Waddell should know, as he was one of the lead authors of a major government report into back ache for the Clinical Standards Advisory Group.[2] 'I'm very much afraid that some of the ways we have handled back pain may actually have made it worse, may have caused more disability than there needs to be.'

Gill is a typical back pain sufferer. Working as a hospital receptionist, she slipped and fell. She went to see her GP, who told her to rest. She did. For over four months she spent most of her day lying on the floor staring at her ceiling, hoping the pain would go. But it didn't. Her GP sent her to the hospital to see a variety of specialists, none of whom could help. This does not surprise Professor Waddell: 'One of the problems is that patients often get sent to see a lot of different medical specialists and the trouble is that most of the specialists that they get sent to see like orthopaedic surgeons and rheumatologists really are not very relevant for ordinary back pain.'

A trip to the hospital also almost always means tests. Every year British doctors send about one and a half million back pain sufferers for X-rays of their spine. Of this one and a half million only 1 per cent have been shown to be relevant to the patient's final treatment. X-rays can even confuse the final diagnosis because they show incidental findings. It is also worth bearing in mind that having an X-ray of the spine involves quite high doses of radiation, about 120 times the amount of radiation that you would receive from a normal chest X-ray. Although the risk for an individual is very low, statistically that increased level of exposure translates into at least nine extra deaths from radiation every year.

WHAT SHOULD I DO?

The message of all the research done on backs over the last ten years is that the best thing to do with a bad back is not to rest it, but to keep it mobile. You either get going or you get disabled. With uncomplicated back ache there is no evidence that activity is harmful or that it will make the pain worse. In fact studies clearly show that keeping going not only stops your back freezing up, but actually reduces pain.[3]

The only time you should take to your bed with uncomplicated back ache is if you are in pain that can't be managed by painkillers and are unable to stand or walk. Even then you should not rest for more than a day or two. If it hasn't improved by then you should see a chartered physiotherapist, a chiropractor or an osteopath. What they all offer is massage and manipulation. Osteopaths and chiropractors, once described by the medical profession as 'unscientific cults', are now regulated and respectable. There is much evidence that skilled massage and manipulation, if done early enough, can make a huge difference and prevent the back ache from becoming chronic. It is important to be treated quickly and properly because once the problem becomes chronic it is much harder to treat.

I keep repeating 'uncomplicated' because there are times when it is vital to get medical help. Consider what happened to a friend of mine, John. He fell down some steps and hurt his back. The pain became more and more excruciating, which was bad, and then he started to develop symptoms. First of all there were tinglings in his legs, then loss of sensation, then he found he couldn't urinate. These are all signs that something was compressing the nerves that run down the spine in the lumbar region, or the small of the back. Compression of the spinal cord requires urgent investigation because unless something is done about it the damage can progress and become permanent. John knew this and went along to his local hospital, where they put him on a trolley, catheterized him, and then left him overnight in casualty. This, as you might gather, is not the right thing to do. Imagine lying there all night knowing that your spinal nerves are being squeezed, that you could be left paralysed or incontinent, and no one is taking it seriously.

John, being an assertive sort of guy, eventually managed to see a consultant neurosurgeon (neurosurgeons are probably a better bet than orthopaedic surgeons if you do need your back operated on; I don't have any concrete evidence to support this view but that is what my medical colleagues tell me). He recognized that it was an emergency and operated immediately. John had a slipped disc which was indeed compressing his spinal nerves; the surgeon sorted it out and this story has a happy ending.

What is really alarming is that the casualty staff did not recognize what was going on. They obviously recognized there was something because they catheterized him, but they didn't make the connection.

HOW TO AVOID IT

I picked up the following tips from a journal on how to avoid straining your back. They are mainly statements of the obvious:

- Try not to trip, stumble or move jerkily

- When lifting a heavy object, bend at the hip and knee rather than bending forward

- Avoid twisting your back

- Don't lift heavy objects at arm's length

- Carry heavy loads symmetrically in front, on the back or on the head.

Back ache is particularly common in parents (of both sexes) and smokers. Another common cause of back pain is bad beds. I am still sleeping in one that I acquired from a friend from medical school who used to make it squeak vigorously every other evening (he is clearly destined for a long life) and this is not a good idea. Apparently you should think about changing your bed every ten years and certainly by the time you and your partner are rolling down into the dip and into each other. According to the National Back Pain Association, buying a bed with a mattress that is really hard and unyielding is as bad for your back as a soft one. A really hard bed will prevent your muscles from relaxing and resting, and as muscles are normally the underlying problem in simple back ache this is not a good idea.

How do you find your perfect bed? I am told the name 'orthopaedic' bed is a bit of a con and means nothing much except that you are paying an awful lot for the bed. The advice from the experts is to try before you buy, which means spending a good half hour or so lying on the bed in the showroom, preferably with your friend, before you decide. Expect funny looks.

For further information contact:
   The National Back Pain Association,
   The Old Office Block, Elm Tree Rd
   Teddington,
   Middlesex
   TW11 8ST
   0181 977 5474

COUGHS AND SNEEZES

We Brits are foolish enough to buy and swallow 6 million gallons of cough mixture a year despite lack of evidence that this money is well spent. As a teenager, I did once drop a Do-Do tablet on the understanding that it had strange mood-altering qualities (I am still waiting) but since then, I can honestly say that not a single drop had passed my lips until recently when I got a tickly cough... I mean really tickly, so tickly that it took over my entire life and plunged me into the depths of despair. I was going to call my family doctor, just for a laugh, and insist that he visit me at home – 'It's too tickly to come to the surgery' – but he has a heart condition and it would probably kill him.

So instead I rang Dr Alan Morice, a consultant respiratory physician in Sheffield, who does research into coughs. He is also deeply sceptical about the benefits of many cough medicines:

'Most coughs are self limiting. With a viral illness you get better by yourself.'

'Alan, I know all that, it's what I tell my patients, but this is a really bad cough. There must be something?'

'The glycerine and sugary type medicines – there is a little bit of evidence that they work. Syrups coat the throat and make you feel better; it's called a demulsant action, so simple syrup works, never mind the cough mixtures with all the drugs in, for which you pay obviously more money. If my children get a dry cough I give them simple linctus; it's cheap and it seems to make them feel better and that's what you want from that type of medicine. It's not going to actually have a pharmacological action, it's more soothing in nature.'

So off I popped to the chemist to browse around the linctuses, but it didn't work. Soon I was back on the phone to Dr Morice who advised me to 'go back to the pharmacy and ask for a strong, centrally acting cough suppressant, and they will be able to advise you.'

Centrally acting drugs act on the cough reflex in the brain and are thought to be the most effective way of suppressing coughs. A number of remedies contain these drugs... but it wasn't really what I fancied. So I pressed Dr Morice on what he himself would take. 'I'm a great believer in honey and lemon. I think that's a very effective remedy, especially with a dash of whisky at night.'

He was right.

THE COMMON COLD

As its name implies, the common cold is one of the commonest illnesses in the world and huge amounts of time, money and research have gone into looking for a cure. It is the holy grail of medical science and whoever finds it is going to be worth billions. I had a patient who used to ring me up and say he had found the cure, but when I asked him what it was, he just said, 'Wouldn't you like to know.'

The reason that no one yet has come close to finding a cure is that there are more than 200 different viruses around that can cause the common cold and these viruses change and mutate all the time, so there is not the remotest chance of a vaccine. Antibiotics only work on bacteria, which is why it's a waste of time and money using them to treat a cold or the flu.

A common belief is that there is some connection between the common cold and being cold. Parents say to children, 'If you don't wrap up well in winter you'll come down with a cold.' But this is a fallacy. If you were to row across the Atlantic naked you wouldn't catch a cold because you need to be exposed to viruses and unless you are exposed to other human beings carrying viruses you will not become infected. The main reason we get so many more colds in winter than in summer is that we tend to huddle together in poorly ventilated buildings, a great breeding ground for illness.

WHO GETS COLDS?

In the UK children average six to eight colds a year and adults two to four. Yet these averages hide a great amount of variability. Only about a third of people who are exposed to common cold viruses actually get a cold. A third shrug it off and the other third carry it, but without symptoms.

In one study, 276 volunteers filled in a questionnaire about their social ties: are you married, do you have children, do you have friends, do you work, are you a member of the local knitting circle? etc. They then had drops containing live rhinoviruses inserted into their nostrils. The researchers then waited to see who would actually get a cold.

Every day the volunteers had their nasal mucus studied, their mucociliary clearance measured, and regular samples taken from their nostrils to see how the viruses were getting on. After a couple of weeks one thing started to become obvious: people with lots of different *types* of social ties were much less likely to catch a cold than the less gregarious, and, if they did, the cold was likely to be less severe. The study showed that 'those with more types of social ties were less susceptible to common colds, produced less mucus, were more effective in ciliary clearance of their nasal passages, and shed less virus.'[4]

In other words they caught milder colds, could blow their noses more effectively and were less likely to pass on viruses. What is funny about this is that it's not so much the number of friends you have that matters but the number of different social groups to which you belong. People with the fewest (one to three) different types of social tie were four times more likely to get a cold than those with the most (six or more) types of social ties. Other factors which *increased* your chances of getting a cold were smoking, sleeping badly, alcohol abstinence (moderate drinkers once again did well), low dietary intake of vitamin C, and being introverted.

So, if you want to avoid getting a cold, get a life. Make more friends, join a club, have some children, go out with your work mates, have a drink, and eat more oranges. Simple.

CAN ANYTHING MAKE IT BETTER?

It is interesting that vitamin C intake was again shown to be a significant factor. As I mentioned earlier, Linus Pauling would have felt vindicated. Pauling was right to believe that vitamin C has a biological effect on the common cold, but he was wildly over-optimistic in how effective it would turn out to be. The trouble was that he based most of his conclusions on a single placebo-controlled trial on schoolchildren in a skiing camp in the Swiss Alps. In this study the children receiving 1 gram of vitamin C a day caught fewer colds and had them for a shorter period of time than those taking placebo. But children in a skiing camp are not exactly representative of the general population and other studies have failed to produce such good results. As I pointed out earlier a meta-analysis of a trial does suggest that taking vitamin C may shorten the duration of your cold, but not whether you get it in the first place. Anyway it's cheap and tasty, and if you believe that taking it will do you good then it probably will.

Zinc

Zinc tablets have recently been hyped as a great treatment for the common cold. There is a scientific rationale behind this: in test tube studies it's been shown that zinc binds to rhinoviruses and stops them from entering human cells. It's a plausible reason for why zinc might help improve your symptoms and even shorten the duration of the disease, but does it work in practice?

In one study 100 patients were given lozenges which contained either 13.3mg of zinc gluconate or placebo and told to suck one every two hours from when they woke up to when they fell asleep.[5] If you are wondering how on earth they manage to persuade people to take part in these sort of trials, well, in this case it was simple: bribery. Patients who finished the study were entered into a raffle where they could win dinner for two or a trip to the Bahamas.

Most colds last about eight days. Our zinc suckers got over their colds in only 4.4 days, while those taking the placebo pills went on sneezing and snuffling for an average of 7.6 days. Zinc clearly seemed to have an effect. The main problem is that you have to take eight lozenges a day and I am told by those who have tried them that they taste vile.

Unfortunately for the fans of zinc, a more recent study in school children came to a rather different conclusion.[6] In children it was considered unethical to deliberately give them a cold, so the researchers had to wait around until they had collected enough kids with signs of an early cold brewing. The 249 children they chose were either given cherry-flavoured lozenges containing 10mg of zinc gluconate which they had to take six times a day for three weeks, or they were given a placebo sugar pill.

The researchers found that children who took the zinc lozenges had their cold symptoms for just as long as those who took the placebo pills. In both groups symptoms lasted an average of nine days. The children who took the zinc lozenges also complained about unpleasant side effects, such as a 'bad taste' in the mouth, nausea, and diarrhoea. The author of this study, Dr Macknin, who had also carried out the previous one in adults, tried to explain why this time it hadn't worked: 'The dosage in our current study may have been too low for children and adolescents. Because the mechanism of action of zinc in treating the common cold is unknown, the optimal dose of medication is also unknown.'

He also speculates that since adults in his earlier study took lemon-lime-flavoured lozenges, and the children took cherry-flavoured ones, it is possible that the cherry flavouring 'in some unknown way inactivated the zinc'. Back to the drawing board for zinc.

Coffee

When I get a stinking cold I pour coffee down my throat until I start to buzz. According to psychologist Dr Andrew Smith of Bristol University

I'm doing just the right thing. Dr Smith tested a hundred volunteers for 'mood and performance' when they were healthy, then asked them to come back when they had caught a cold. Sneezing away, they were then re-tested before and after drinking fruit juice, decaffeinated coffee and ordinary coffee. The tests consisted of getting the volunteers to rate their mood, then do reaction tests. The idea of the fruit juice and the decaff was to act as a control, to see if it might just be taking lots of fluid that made a difference.

Anyway, what he found was that having a cold makes you less alert, less efficient and more miserable. No surprises there. He also found that drinking fruit juice and decaffeinated coffee didn't do much to help, but that coffee with caffeine restored the poor suffering cold victims to pretty much the same mental state they were in when they were healthy. Good news for coffee drinkers, and for the coffee industry who supported this research.

The Best Treatment
According to Dr Ron Eccles who runs the Common Cold Research Centre at Cardiff University, the best thing you can do for a cold is the sort of thing I'm sure your mother told you:

- Get plenty of bed rest and drink lots of fluids

- If you have a sort throat try gargling with warm salt water or soluble aspirin

- Take aspirin or paracetamol to reduce the headaches and the feeling of chilliness you get with a cold

My own advice is not to go to your doctor unless you are really ill because:

- That is all they're going to say

- It might be me

- Sitting around in surgeries means you are likely to give someone else your cold or pick up a new one instead

HOW DO I AVOID GETTING ONE?

A few years back a tissue manufacturer tried selling tissues impregnated with an anti-viral chemical. The only problem was that the tissues didn't stop you getting a cold, they just decreased the chance you would give your cold to someone else. The tissues did not sell. The advice from the American Medical Association on how to avoid a cold is simple:

● Wash your hands frequently

● Don't touch your nose or eyes after coming in contact with a person with a cold

The reason for this advice is that one of the main ways you get a cold is not from people sneezing in your face, but from your own hands. What happens is that they sneeze, wipe their hands on their snotty noses, shake your hand and so transfer the virus. You then inject the virus into yourself, either by sticking your finger up your nose or by rubbing your eyes. It is almost impossible not to do it, which is why a trip to the bathroom after meeting someone with a red nose is advisable.

ANXIETY AND DEPRESSION

'Depression is contagious,' a depressed psychiatrist told me on his retirement. It is a theory which may have some substance to it (in Germany there is a trial going on at the moment, treating depressed patients with anti-viral drugs) but it is not one you will hear many psychiatrists pushing. As my friend Matthew assured me, 'Surrounding yourself with mental illness is very stressful and can precipitate depression in those who are disposed to it, but it doesn't cause it.' He then regaled me with his theory of depression ('it's a result of altered receptor sensitivity to mono-amine transmitters in certain areas of the brain') with all the enthusiasm of someone who has become a consultant at the tender age of thirty-two.

The explanation of mental illnesses in biochemical terms has given psychiatry some scientific credibility, but being depressed is still not seen as the equivalent of having a broken leg. The myth persists that mental illness is incurable and that all psychiatrists are mad, depressed and bearded (which some, of course, are). As I mentioned earlier, even doctors are wary of admitting to being depressed because of the stigma and risk to their careers. I know only two hospital doctors, both psychiatrists, who have spoken openly about their depression and both waited until they were consultants to do it. One visited a consultant outside his area, had a course of electro-convulsive therapy and is now much better. The other is counting off the days to a mood-enhancing retirement.

WHAT IS IT?

If you are tearful for no apparent reason, pessimistic about the future, feel negative about yourself and guilty about the past then you may well be depressed. You are also likely to be a woman, because men, although they also become depressed, are more likely to express their depression by drinking more, working harder, jogging obsessively or getting into fights. It will affect a quarter of us as some point in our lives and it is on the increase. Although it can be triggered by losing your job or the death of someone close, it can also come out of the blue. I regularly see patients who say, 'I've never felt like this before, and I don't understand why.'

Professor Lewis Wolpert has not only studied and written about depression and its treatments, he has also experienced it: 'I stopped going to work, felt terrible. In fact I can't even remember the details now, it's quite odd… I started taking sleeping pills. Then one night at about four o'clock in the morning I woke up with an overwhelming compulsion to commit suicide.'

Professor Wolpert did what I would do in his circumstances; he started on a short course of antidepressants and combined this with a talking treatment called cognitive behavioural therapy.

DRUGS

Antidepressant drugs are the commonest way of treating depression, whether it comes out of the blue or is precipitated by a crisis in your life. They can be very effective – at least in the short term – but patients do not like taking them and GPs, even when they make the right diagnosis, often give too small a dose for too short a time. You will commonly be prescribed tricyclic antidepressants or selective serotonin re-uptake inhibitors (SSRIs), of which the best known is Prozac. Both classes of drugs can have unpleasant side-effects and the SSRIs can also, paradoxically, make anxiety worse. Why American psychiatrists are handing it out like candy is a mystery to me, because one of Prozac's well-recognized side-effects is that it can dampen sexual drive. As an ironic contrast, in one study they gave the wives of men on Prozac a stop-watch to measure 'delay to orgasm', another unfortunate side effect of the drug.

The biggest problem with a drug-only approach is that there tends to be a high relapse rate when people stop taking them. In one study the doctors randomly allocated patients to either receiving drugs, drugs plus cognitive behavioural therapy (CBT) or CBT alone.[7] Two years down the road and 78 per cent of patients given drugs alone had had a relapse or recurrence of their illness. Patients receiving cognitive therapy and drugs, or cognitive therapy alone, did far better, with a relapse rate of only 21 per cent and 23 per cent respectively.

TALKING THERAPIES

There are two quite different Big Ideas in psychotherapy. The best known is the one based on the works of Sigmund Freud: psychoanalysis. Central to psychoanalysis is the belief that current mental illness is the result of unconscious conflicts and the way to recover is to bring them to the surface and resolve them. From the first there has been little attempt to prove any of these claims. Freud himself relied on anecdotes (which he called 'case studies') and was not above claiming successes where failure would be a more accurate description.

For example, one of the first 'successes' attributed to psychoanalysis was the case of 'Anna O'. 'Anna' was a girl of twenty-one who, while nursing her sick father, became ill. She developed first a cough and then other, more bizarre symptoms. She complained of troubles with her vision, unpredictable fits and strange outbursts. She was labelled as a case of hysteria and treated with the new talking therapy. According to a paper published in 1895 by Freud and Breurer (the GP who treated her) psychoanalysis helped resolve her symptoms and she was cured.

Later the true story emerged. Freud's official biographer revealed that 'Anna O' was a woman called Bertha Pappenheim. When her medical records were tracked down it was obvious that Bertha had contracted tubercular meningitis from her father, who had died of it. Her symptoms were almost certainly caused by that disease, not by hysteria. Far from being cured by psychoanalysis, shortly after her 'treatment' she was admitted to a sanatorium in a terrible state. There she slowly recovered under conventional medical care.

DOES IT WORK?

Psychoanalysis has provided psychiatry with valuable insights, but is an impractical form of therapy because it is so expensive and time consuming. There is also no convincing evidence that it is an effective treatment for depression. The people who are the most likely to get something out of it are YAVISes, those who are Young, Attractive, Verbal, Intelligent, Successful. This may explain why it is so attractive to artists, students, intellectuals and Hollywood script writers. Before starting on psychoanalysis you should be warned that it may not make you better and may make you worse.

BEHAVIOURAL THERAPIES

The other main type of psychotherapy is based on the behaviourist tradition, which started with a Russian, Ivan Pavlov. He showed that if you ring a bell just before giving a dog its food, then the dog will come to associate the sound of the bell with eating. The dog will soon salivate just on hearing the bell. Pavlov suggested that humans also respond to reward and punishment by association, and that these associations can dominate our lives. The idea that we, like other animals, are partly the product of conditioning is less flattering than the idea that we are the product of complex interactions between our Id, Ego and Superego. The behaviourist approach, however, has produced far more useful and effective treatments for a range of mental illnesses.

One example is phobias. Perhaps you have a phobia about spiders so that every time you see them you feel fear: your heart pounds, you feel sick. The fear is completely out of proportion to the actual danger, but that is no longer the point. Soon even thinking about them can trigger the reaction; you have been conditioned to associate spiders with fear. Psychoanalysts would go hunting for the cause, the thing that originally triggered the fear. Freud, for example, tried to treat a little boy called Hans with a horse phobia by telling him (via his father) that he was afraid of the horse because the horse had a large penis, like his father's. This may or may not have been true, but it certainly wasn't helpful. A behaviourist would say, forget the cause, change the associations. Teach little Hans to associate horses with pleasure, not terror. Reward him for patting the horse, read him stories about friendly horses, for instance. Phobias respond very well to this sort of treatment, known as desensitization.

Cognitive Behavioural Therapy

The biggest advance in the treatment of depression in recent years has been the development of cognitive behavioural therapy (CBT). Crudely, the difference between behaviourists and CBT is that while behaviourists change the way you feel by changing the way you behave, cognitive therapists change the way you feel by changing the way you think.

Funnily enough, the man credited with CBT's early development was a Freudian analyst, Aaron Beck. He says he first had the idea while listening to one of his patients describing a sexual encounter. He noticed that as she was speaking she was becoming more and more anxious. Beck assumed this was because she was talking about sex, but when he probed more deeply it was clear something else was going on. She told Beck that while she was talking to him she kept thinking, 'He doesn't like me; he's bored with me.' It was these thoughts that were making her anxious.

It is now clear that most people who are depressed have negative automatic thoughts (NATs), thoughts that flash in and out of their minds. These thoughts are destructive and seem to have a life of their own, like an evil genie on your shoulder. You're walking down the street and wave to a friend, but he does not respond. The genie whispers, 'The reason he ignored you is because he doesn't like you, nobody ever has, you're repellent.' Such thoughts naturally make you feel low and more depressed and increase the likelihood that you will have further negative automatic thoughts.

Cognitive therapists do not claim that this sort of negative thinking causes depression in the first place, but they do claim that NATs help keep you depressed long after the original triggering event has gone. So, amongst other things, a cognitive therapist will challenge negative lines of thinking and encourage the person to come up with more reasonable and positive interpretations such as, 'The reason they ignored me is because they didn't see me'. Patients are also encouraged to rate their anxieties on a scale of one to ten, and to control them with relaxation techniques. It sounds ludicrously simple, but research shows it is very effective. A recent review of fifteen different studies concluded that CBT was at least as effective at treating depressed patients as drugs in the short term, that it worked better in the long term, and that combining the two treatments was more effective than using either one alone.

Therapy consists of between six and twenty one-hour sessions, all aimed at helping you learn to take control of your own thoughts and stamp out your NATs.

CBT has also been shown to be highly effective at treating a huge range of mental disorders ranging from anxiety to the management of sex offenders.[8] The really sad thing is that, despite the fact that CBT is one of the few psychological interventions that really does work, there are still not many trained cognitive behaviour therapists around.

FURTHER INFORMATION

For fact sheets on cognitive behavioural therapy for depression or anxiety send a stamped addressed envelope (stating which disorder you want details about) to:

British Association for Behavioural and Cognitive Therapy
PO Box 9, Accrington
Lancashire BB5 2GD
http://www.gallaudet.edu/~11mgourn/cbt.html

BOOKS
Staying Sane Dr Raj Persaud (Metro Books, 1998)
Overcoming Anxiety Helen Kennerly (Robinson, 1997)
The Freudian Fallacy E.M. Thornton (Thornton, 1985)

SOCIETIES
UK Council for Psychotherapy
167–169 Great Portland Street, London W1N 5FB
Tel 0171 436 3002
Fax 0171 436 3013

MIND, The National Association for Mental Health
Granta House, 15–19 Broadway
Stratford, London E15 4BQ

OBESITY

I once worked for a consultant once who was as thin as a rake and who had no time at all for patients who claimed they were fat and getting fatter despite only eating a lettuce leaf every other day. 'There were no fat people in Belsen,' he would bark before suggesting some particularly rigorous diet.

Any number of scientific studies have revealed the same cruel truth, that obesity has nothing to do with big bones and everything to do with how much you eat and how much energy you burn off. Many of these studies have been done in a 'metabolic chamber', small rooms where volunteers stay for a week at a time. Here they are fed normal meals, but every gram of everything that they eat is measured to assess its energy content. The researchers also check exactly how much energy the volunteers' bodies burn off when they are doing a range of activities (there are a number of complex ways of doing this that involve explaining concepts like isotopes, which I'd simply rather not do). The conclusion of all these studies is that overweight people eat more and burn up their food *faster* than thin people.

When fat people run for a bus they will use up more energy than thin people simply because of their bigger bodyweight. Asleep or at work, their bodies will be consuming energy faster than their less horizontally challenged colleagues, and this is why dieting is so hard. The typical pattern of a dieter is that you cut down what you eat and you start to lose weight. But as your weight drops you burn off less energy getting around. Unless you compensate by doing more exercise, you will find that although you are eating less and feeling ravenously hungry most of the time, you are not losing any more weight. You become depressed, go back to your old habits and pile on the pounds. This helps explain why, despite the fact that we spend at least £1 billion a year on diets, 90 per cent of slimmers will within a year have put back on at least as much weight as they originally lost.

Experimentally this has been demonstrated by Rudolph Leibel, a nutritionist. He did an eight-year study of eighteen obese patients and twenty-three lean ones. Every so often they would come along to his lab and for three months at a time have themselves intensely monitored, everything from what they ate to the calorie content of what they excreted. He found that lean and obese people respond to weight gain or weight loss in exactly the same way, by trying to return to their starting point. When his patients put on weight, their bodies compensated by burning more energy; when they lost weight, their bodies responded by consuming less.[9]

It is because our bodies like to keep to a set point that people who just diet are almost certainly doomed to fail. The only way out of this dilemma is to forget calorie counting and get on your bike, because what is now blindingly obvious is that the real reason for the surge in obesity over the last few decades is not that we are eating more but that we are doing less.

The average Briton is consuming about a third fewer calories than twenty years ago, yet there are now twice as many obese people around as there were then. It is not just that we can't be bothered to walk upstairs or run for the bus, although that is certainly true, but also that everything at home is geared to ensuring minimal effort. The Dunn Clinical Nutrition Centre in Cambridge, which carries out research into energy consumption, has come up with figures which make surprising reading:

- If you stop using a cordless phone you'll increase the amount you walk around the house by about 10 miles a year

- Making a bed uses up 15,000 more calories a year than simply flinging on the duvet

- A shopping trip thirty years ago was done largely on foot and would have burnt off 2,400 calories. The same trip today, done by car, would use 280 calories

- Abandon the television remote control and you'll walk three miles more a year

Of all our leisure activities, watching the television is (metabolically speaking) the closest to death. The average Briton spends about four hours a day watching TV, while in the United States, where obesity is much worse, they watch an average of about seven hours a day. If you spent that twenty-eight hours a week doing something else, like walking or gardening, you would burn off an additional 4,200 calories a week, the equivalent of two days' food.

When it comes to children things are as bad, if not worse. The average British child is carrying about 1.5kg more fat than their parents were at the same age and children are now astonishingly slothful. In 1985 children under fifteen walked an average of 247 miles a year. By 1993 they were walking less than 198 miles. Over the same time period they also cut back on cycling, down from 38 miles a year to 29.[10] And girls are worse than boys; apparently the average teenage girl is physically active (the equivalent of walking) for less than fifteen minutes a day, and that includes PE lessons at school.

One reason children are doing less exercise these days is because they are being driven to school. Walking to school used to account for almost half the walking children did. Parents are being urged to encourage their children to walk to school on the grounds that it is good for them, but the trouble is that this is not necessarily true. As the *Lancet* points out if you are a child under fifteen you are fifty times more likely to be killed walking to school than being driven (4.8 deaths against 0.1 deaths per 100 million miles travelled).[11] The chance of being killed either way is small, but real. And what is truly ironic is that in making the 'safe' choice to drive your children to school, you are increasing traffic volume and therefore increasing the risk to the few remaining kids who are walking.

TIPS TO AVOID OBESITY

- Drink at least six glasses of ice-cold water a day; people sometimes confuse thirst for hunger. Water will also fill you up and you will consume energy heating it up. Low-calorie drinks are no substitute because they contain artificial sweeteners. These may not have any calories, but they trick your body into thinking it is taking in sugar, so your blood sugar levels fall in preparation for the sugar onslaught. But when no sugar arrives you end up feeling hungrier than before.

- Replace fat in your diet with carbohydrate and starch. In other words, eat as much bread, rice and potatoes as you want, just don't drown them in butter and oil. One reason for this is that fat is very dense in energy with 1 gram of butter containing twice as many calories as a gram of bread. But just as bad is the fact that eating a fatty meal does not stop you feeling hungry; it isn't anything like as good an appetite suppressant as carbohydrate or protein. Your body can only store about 900g of carbohydrate before it shouts, 'I'm full'. We have, however, an almost infinite capacity for storing fat.

All this is true, but it may seem fairly obvious. There are a few scientists out there pursuing more off-the-wall solutions, such as the researcher who has shown that chewing each mouthful for five minutes stimulates an area of the brain called the secondary taste cortex, which in turn makes you feel full, or those researchers who are trying to prove that obesity is catching – Nikil Dhurandhar and Richard Atkinson of the University of

Wisconsin Medical School in the USA have reported finding antibodies to a virus known as AD-36 in 23 out of 154 volunteers that they recruited from a weight loss centre. This adenovirus is known to cause coughs and colds in humans, but apparently also causes obesity in chickens. Studies have apparently shown that despite eating the same amount of food as fellow birds, chickens infected with this virus put on more weight and were less inclined to do exercise.

PAIN

If you experienced crippling pain following an illness, operation or accident, you might expect someone to sort it out. Certainly, we have the knowledge and the technology. As Dr Douglas Justins, a consultant anaesthetist and pain management specialist at London's St Thomas's Hospital puts it: 'In this day and age it's totally unacceptable for anyone still to be suffering acute pain in a hospital.'

An Audit Commission Report, *Anaesthesia under Examination*, found that the experiences of patients going into different hospitals varied widely. In some hospitals 90 per cent of patients said they were left in moderate to severe pain, while in others this figure was down to 10 per cent. Although many trusts have barely enough anaesthetists to put people to sleep, let alone run pain clinics, in my experience the way pain is handled has a lot to do with the attitudes of the staff. The way to obtain pain relief is to demand it, not just lie back and groan.

I remember being called out by a nurse in the middle of the night, 'because one of the patients has gone mad'. He was a post-operative patient who was in a corner of the room swinging his catheter with dangerously full urine bag around his head. 'Should we call the psychiatrists?' she asked. It was 3a.m. so I went over and asked if he was OK. 'Yes,' the patient replied, 'it's just that I have this terrible pain. I'd like something to soothe it, and rather than shout and wake up these other folk I thought I'd get her attention.'

At undergraduate level, training in pain management is often pitiful, and many health professionals qualify with quaintly stoical views about pain and a reticence to use opiod pain-killers. Morphine is a brilliant painkiller and has been used for centuries, and yet many doctors either refuse to give it or don't give enough for fear of overdosing or causing addiction. This is perhaps why half of all cancer patients and a third of cardiac patients suffer constant, unnecessary pain. Dr Douglas

Justins says this is absurd: 'The reluctance to prescribe morphine is a long-standing problem based on tradition, misconceptions, misinformation and a lack of education. It is perceived as a very dangerous drug.'

In fact, even when patients are on large doses to control their pain, the chances of becoming a drug addict are 'infinitesimally small'. It's more likely for pain to kick in because a doctor is reluctant to increase the dose. Unfortunately the public shares these beliefs about opiods and assume that when a doctor gives morphine he or she is trying to finish them off. So the best pain relief we have remains misunderstood and underused, as roofer Rod Buck can testify:

> I fell 30 feet off a roof and landed on my back. I broke most of my ribs and the broken ends penetrated the lungs... In intensive care, the pain was overwhelming. It was out of this world, it actually paralysed me, I couldn't move, all my muscles clamped up and I was absolutely frozen rigid.

After two weeks of pain and forceful complaining, Rod got what he needed:

> I was rescued by an anaesthetic consultant who had a special interest in pain management and prescribed morphine for me. But once I was on the general wards, I was aware of a subtle disapproval on the part of many of the staff of me being on morphine, rather as if I was a sort of an alcoholic or child molester, certainly a person of weak moral fibre, because I was needing to take this stuff. However, I persisted, demanded and got adequate analgesia. I think a lot of people give up in the face of determined opposition of the nursing and junior medical staff.

For less severe pain there are plenty of other drugs available, and if the one prescribed isn't working, ask for another. The following were recommended to me by a pain expert:

> Mild pain: Paracetamol 1,000 mg four times a day
> Moderate pain: Co-codamol (which normally consists of codeine phosphate 8mg plus paracetamol 500mg) one or two tablets four times a day
> Severe pain: Co-codamol one or two tablets four times a day plus naproxen 500 mg twice a day

For people with chronic pain who don't want to take drugs there is acupuncture (discussed in the next chapter) and also transcutaneous electrical nerve stimulation (TENS), which is widely used. There is also a curious alternative that I only recently came across, capsaicin cream, a cream based on chillies.

THE CHILLI TREATMENT

The mysterious thing about chillies is that, as well as causing pain, they can relieve it. The practice of using chillies to treat pain was popular back in the fifteenth century and although it is not something modern doctors have bothered themselves with much, chillies are now making a modest come-back in the form of pain-relieving creams. The active ingredient in chilli first stimulates then prevents the production of a pain-transmitting chemical called 'substance P' in the pain fibres. No more P, no more pain.

When Joy developed an inflammation of the tendons in her hand she was left in agony following an operation. Then she went to a pain clinic where she was prescribed a chilli cream to rub along the scar-line. 'I can wear sleeves now and touch the back of my hand whereas I couldn't before. They felt like barbed wire if they touched my skin because my skin was always super-sensitive, but now I can wear them with no problem.'

A study in the *European Journal of Clinical Pharmacology* reviewed the evidence for the effectiveness of the cream in a range of conditions.[12] The patients rubbed in the cream several times a day for several weeks. It worked for some things better than others:

Diabetic neuropathy
73 per cent of patients had their pain relieved by capsaicin compared with 49 per cent of patients given placebo

Osteoarthritis
45 per cent of patients improved with capsaicin compared with 16 per cent with placebo

Postmastectomy pain
Using the cream four times a day for six weeks produced pain relief in 38 per cent of patients with capsaicin compared with 10 per cent of patients with placebo

The main advantage of capsaicin cream is that it is selective, works just on the painful fibres, and avoids the drowsiness, stomach problems and constipation that are sometimes associated with powerful pain-killing drugs. But what is also very striking about these studies is how effective the placebo creams were. Now if only I could prescribe them ...

FURTHER INFORMATION

For more on capsaicin cream (also known as Axsain) ask your GP or contact the manufacturers (Bioglan Pharmaceuticals 01462 438444).

For details of your nearest local pain clinic contact:
> The Pain Society,
> 9 Bedford Square,
> London WC1B 3RA
> Tel: 0171 636 2750

10 | THE ALTERNATIVES

Richard Asher, a distinguished London physician, was spot on when he observed: 'The success of a therapy depends as much on the enthusiasm of the therapist as the faith of the patient. If you fervently believe in your treatment, even if controlled trials show it is quite useless, your results are much better, your patients are much better and your income is much better too.'

Certainly one of the reasons complementary medicines are so popular is that their practitioners have more time, more belief in what they're doing and often more compassion than doctors. It's a tough choice. Do you favour Ralph the holistic healer with his thirty minutes of unconditional therapeutic touch, or Dr Bates, the lonely, divorced, alcoholic bigot with his five minutes of medically approved cynicism? At least Dr Bates's time always comes free.

Some complementary practitioners – osteopaths and chiropractors – have made a determined effort to prove their worth and become properly regulated. Rather than fight the orthodoxy, they decided to become part of it. Once they had shown in proper clinical trials that they were rather better at treating backs than conventional doctors they were grudgingly admitted to the mainstream. Other complementary medicines, such as homeopathy, acupuncture and faith healing, have put themselves to the test with mixed results (more on them later). Most, however, remain completely unregulated and very much a case of 'buyer beware'.

I have a soft spot for 'alternatives' and have tried out a number of them, ranging from being hung upside down between the thighs of a mystic on a Welsh mountain to being rubbed all over by a bearded enthusiast in a swimming pool. They have mostly been enjoyable experiences, if not necessarily life-enhancing. The one that struck me as being strictly for those who are soft in the head is radionics. Does anyone who has more than two neurones to rub together really believe that by dowsing a lump of excrement with a pendulum and plugging the results into an electronic box it is possible to figure out your physical, emotional and spiritual well-being, as well as your risk of getting AIDS, diabetes and cancer? Who would part with a thousand pounds for a computer program and a black box containing a few wires just because they are told that twiddling the knobs will reduce their risk of developing these diseases? I decided I had to find out.

First I watched a patient, Imogen, being plugged into the Automated Computer Treatment System which 'conducts a two-way flow of bio-energetic information between the patient's body and a data base of over 260,000 different energy treatments'. Imogen loved it:

> After two minutes I was aware of a large circular globe of energy from about my navel to about my forehead, which gradually contracted down and focused very strongly on my throat. After a while, the energy slid up to my third eye and circled round in an anti-clockwise direction... I've never experienced anything like that; very impressive.

With a build-up like that I couldn't wait for my turn, but I felt nothing. My third eye refused to be energized. Gordon, my therapist, was not surprised. 'It seems to have more of an effect in women,' he observed.

Gordon really believes in what he's doing, and his belief in radionics is unshakeable. Unfortunately, his black boxes are not. Inside is a seemingly random collection of inductors and capacitors, some not connected up at all and some short circuiting each other. I asked him how it worked. 'Radionics is easily explained in terms of quantum physics. All matter produces energy fields that can be manipulated – I can treat animals, plants, crops and soil.'

A little probing revealed that Gordon knows little about quantum physics, so next he admitted: 'I'm not exactly sure how it works but I don't really mind as long as it does – a bit like my car, really.'

All in all I had an enjoyable day out and a good laugh, and since laughter is supposed to be therapeutic, I suppose I was better for the experience. But if radionics is a joke, what about the top three most popular complementary medicines in Britain: homeopathy, acupuncture, healing?

HOMEOPATHY

Homoeopathy was invented in the eighteenth century by Samuel Hahnemann. He was appalled by the blood-letting, emetics and purges that went by the name of medicine in those days. He came up with the not unreasonable idea that the body has an amazing capacity to heal itself and should be encouraged to do so. But then he came off the rails, or perhaps just took his train off on a different track.

First of all he decided that 'like cures like', for example if you have a patient with a runny nose you give them red onion extract to make the runny nose runnier.

Next he came up with the concept of 'minimum dilutions', the idea being that homeopathic medicines work best when they are very dilute. This is just as well because homeopaths put into their potions substances such as arsenic, wolf spiders and deadly nightshade that would be lethal at full strength (a homeopath once gave me *nux vomica* – otherwise known as strychnine, a rather unpleasant poison – as a treatment for stress). This idea, that the weaker the solution the stronger the effect, really irritates scientists. If something is diluted with water up to 100 times, as is common in homeopathic preparations, the chance that there is any trace of the original substance left is somewhere between remote and non-existent. You would need to drink about 800,000 gallons of some homeopathic preparations to have a reasonable chance of swallowing a single active molecule. Homeopaths claim that the water somehow 'remembers' what was put in it. Peter Fisher, Medical Director of the Royal London Homeopathic Hospital, offered me an explanation, or at least an analogy:

> If you take a homeopathic medicine to an analytical chemist and say, 'What's in here?' you're quite right, he will say, 'Water, sucrose, and maybe a bit of alcohol', because that's what it's made up in, but if you take that same analytical chemist a floppy disk and say, 'What's in here?' he will say, 'Vinyl and ferric oxide'. Yet for all he knows it might contain the complete works of Shakespeare. Water retains information, retains the memory of something that it's been in contact with, rather like a floppy disk.

So what is the evidence that it actually works? Dr Fisher is able to point to at least two trials in a hyper-respectable journal, the *Lancet*.[1]

Dr David Reilly, a conventionally trained GP who works at the Glasgow Homeopathic hospital tested a homeopathic treatment on twenty-eight volunteers with hay fever or allergic asthma. Those with hay fever received pills made up from grass pollen on the principle of 'like cures like' and the asthmatics received pills made from cat fur, bed-bug mites, whatever their poison was. Half had placebo pills, and no one knew what they were getting. They were all then sent off to see how they did.

Infuriatingly for the sceptics, the homeopathic preparations outperformed the placebo. Not very impressively, but they did it. This left the editors of the *Lancet* scratching their heads. They decided to publish, but put in a rider: 'The dilution principle of homeopathy is absurd…but carefully done work of this sort should not be denied the attention of *Lancet* readers.'

A really impressive result would have been if someone else had carried out a similar trial and secured a similar response, demonstrating that it wasn't just good luck. Unfortunately they haven't. What someone has done is get together all the decent trials they could find on homeopathy and see what they add up to.[2] They were pretty systematic: 'We sought studies from computerized bibliographies and contacts with researchers, institutions, manufacturers, individual collectors, homeopathic conference proceedings and books. We included all languages.'

They found eighty-nine different trials, conducted in everything from allergies to surgery and anaesthesia. In thirty-seven of the trials homeopathy outperformed placebo, in fifty-two of the trials it didn't. In most of the studies the effects were marginal, though there was one area where the results for homeopathy really did seem to come through, in something called postoperative ileus.

Postoperative ileus is when your bowel seizes up after an operation. The researchers found seven trials involving hundreds of patients. The homeopathic treatments used were derived mainly from opium (the idea being that since opium clogs you up, dilute opium will purge you). The way they'd measured success or failure in these trials was by timing how soon after an operation patients either farted ('time to first flatus') or popped off to the loo ('time to first faeces').

What the trials showed was that, on average, the time to first flatus was cut by an impressive 7.4 hours in the people taking homeopathic remedies. So chalk up a major victory for homeopathy? Yes and no. Unfortunately, in the largest study there was no difference between homeopathy and placebo, while the studies that used the most dilute potions (and which, according to the homeopaths, should have been the strongest) had the least effect. All in all it leaves me wondering why homeopaths haven't managed to assemble more proof that it works after 200 years of treating patients.

Conspiracy fans believe that proper trials are not being done because if ten-a-penny homeopathy remedies were shown to be as effective as stuffing your nose with expensive steroids, the medical establishment would be mightily aggrieved. Certainly, the treatments for which we have sound scientific proofs tend to be those for which the drug industry has stumped up billions. When they find one that works, they do not want some homeopath coming along with his *nux vomica* and taking their business.

There are also homeopaths who don't want their trade sent through the scientific mincing machine. They argue that each treatment is tailored to the individual: no two people are alike and each remedy is carefully matched not just to symptoms (*particulars*) but habits (*generals*) and personality traits (*mentals*). A jolly fat woman with itchy lumps would get a different remedy to a thin neurotic one. Hence the scientific habit of treating all itchy-lumped people the same won't work for homeopathy. This attitude amounts to saying, 'Blessed are those who believe without any proof.'

I would love to believe that homeopathy works, then I could prescribe its remedies with conviction and save the NHS a fortune. Certainly, swallowing a sugar tablet that has been doused in water and shaken in a special way is less likely to harm you than unnecessary X-rays or antibiotics. I had just started trying hard to believe when I met a man who'd been to the Royal London Homeopathic Hospital and been given, amongst other things, an infinitesimally dilute solution of the Berlin Wall to unite his disparate symptoms. Needless to say, the patient was delighted. 'Those itchy lumps have gone for good...'

ACUPUNCTURE

When I was a senior house officer, a junior doctor came back from a weekend course on acupuncture with ten packets of needles and a textbook. He had the nerve to try it out in the Geriatric Day Unit with the book open for reference on his lap. For maximum placebo effect, he used the traditional names of the acupuncture points rather than the numbers: 'I'm just trying to find your Encircling Glory, Mrs Fanshaw...' and so on.

He was, of course, extremely popular with elderly patients starved of attention, conversation and touch. One of the consultants was so impressed that he borrowed the textbook and started acupuncture without even bothering with the course. I suppose, though, that this frighteningly slapdash approach is not far removed from conventional medical training – there are plenty of doctors who learned to do lumbar punctures or put in chest drains or take liver biopsies with the textbook open on their knees. As you'll remember from Chapter 2, 86 per cent of surgeons have done operations for the first time alone and unsupervised.

But is it vital to learn the lingo, master the mugwort and suss out the where and whys before getting stuck in? I have read enough to know that traditional acupuncturists believe that a person's health is dependent upon the balance of energy which flows through the body in energy channels and that these energy lines do not fit in with any nerve pathways that have been mapped by Western anatomists. This does not worry practitioners such as anaesthetist Dr George Ghaly: 'There are theories: release of certain substances that could affect the centre in the brain that controls nausea and vomiting. I don't think this is very important. I've been doing anaesthetics for more 25 years and if you ask me how anaesthetics works, I don't know. Nobody knows.'

Dr Ghaly started out as a sceptic about acupuncture, and did some research. His particular interest is in the nausea that many patients experience after an operation. He had heard acupuncturists claim that five minutes of twiddling with a needle in the P6 point (a point situated between the tendons on the inside of the wrist) helps control nausea and vomiting, so he tried it. He did a double-blind, randomized, controlled trial of acupuncture versus placebo in 81 patients.[3] The results were impressive: only one-third of the patients who'd had acupuncture felt nauseous after their operation compared to two-thirds who had received placebo.

As a sceptic I was quite ready to dismiss this as a one-off study. However, this study is just one of many that have come to the same conclusion.

Dr Andrew Vickers is employed by the Research Council for Complementary Medicine (a well-respected body, funded by the European Community) to spend his days assessing and generally ripping into what passes for research amongst fans of complementary medicine. He is particularly unimpressed by the extravagant claims coming out of the East: 'If you look at China or Japan or Taiwan, it doesn't matter what the study's on, acupuncture always works, so this suggests that maybe they will only publish the research if it's positive and that's grounds for caution.'

Dr Vickers says many acupuncture claims have failed when put to a rigorous test in the West. Does acupuncture help smokers stop smoking? Yes, it does, but it is no better than sham acupuncture (where you stick a needle into a part of the body that is well away from any established acupuncture point) and the effect seems to wear off very fast. However, when it comes to controlling nausea and vomiting, Andrew Vickers says that the P6 point has come through in most trials: 'If you just look at the thirteen or fourteen best trials – these were double-blinds, placebo-controlled, randomized trials – most of those trials did show that acupuncture had an effect on nausea and vomiting that could not be explained by placebo.'

This is not perhaps the most clear-cut, ringing endorsement that you would like to hear as a practitioner approaches you with needle at the ready, but I am nevertheless impressed. A drug-free way of controlling nausea would be very useful, particularly the nausea associated with pregnancy. Morning sickness, I am told, is like floating out at sea in a force three gale on a giant rubber duck after having drunk far too much the night before. Doctors used to be free with the prescription pad when women came in complaining of morning sickness, until they discovered that one of their more effective treatments, Thalidomide, was doing more than making women feel less queasy. Ever since Thalidomide women have been understandably anxious about taking drugs during pregnancy, and since acupuncture seems to be side-effect free (just make sure the person doing it is using sterile needles) it sounds like a great boon.

I have only met one woman who has actually tried it for morning sickness. Tracy started out by saying that there was no way someone was going to turn her into a pin cushion, but in the end the endless vomiting got to her and she decided to give it a go. She was quite impressed: 'I had acupuncture once a week after that and it didn't cure it but it actually has eased the sickness for me and made my life a lot easier.'

Research is going on into other areas where acupuncture may have something to contribute over and above placebo, the control of pain being an important one. A problem they've all encountered is sorting out 'placebo' acupuncture effects from 'real' ones. As Professor Ernst of the Department of Complementary Medicine at Exeter University comments when talking about trials on its use in osteoarthritis:

The most rigorous studies suggest that acupuncture is not superior to sham-needling in reducing the pain of osteoarthritis: both alleviate symptoms to roughly the same degree. This could either mean sham-needling has similar specific effects as acupuncture or that both methods are associated with considerable non-specific effects.

At a practical level I don't care too much whether my patients are getting relief as a result of a sham or a real effect. However, I can't see acupuncture becoming an important part of mainstream NHS practice for the more mundane reason that it takes so much time. The only occasion I've ever consulted an acupuncturist, he took half an hour to assess me before reaching for his needles and the needles stayed in for a good fifteen minutes. I have a GP friend, Bob, who told me how he'd tried acupuncture on his arthritis patients with pleasing results: 'I loved the novelty value, they felt they were getting something special and I didn't have to dish out the painkillers.'

So is he still doing it?

> No. I thought I could sort them out with a few treatments, but they kept coming back again and again, and I just got fed up with prattling on about meridians and Qi when in my heart I think it's rubbish. I had to put on an act every time and it got quite tiring. So now they're all back to three months' worth of Brufen and a pat on the back.

You're better off finding someone who has time and really believes. For details see the end of the chapter.

FAITH HEALING

Loving, caring, being part of a community, these are the sort of things that science has been poor at evaluating and yet they contribute far more to our health and sense of well-being than any number of drugs are likely to. Although there have been few studies that have set out to measure the effects of love, there have been some which show graphically the effects of not being loved. One of the most impressive was done unintentionally in post-war Germany.[4]

In this study they looked at children growing up in two orphanages. The orphanages were quite close to each other and the children were, thanks to rationing, getting identical amounts of food. In the Bienenhaus orphanage the children suffered under the tyranny of the stern and forbidding Fraulein Schwarz. The children in this orphanage put on less weight and grew less quickly than children in the nearby Volgenest orphanage cared for by the affectionate and warm-hearted Fraulein Grun. Then, part way through the study, the grim Fraulein Schwarz replaced the affectionate Fraulein Grun at the Volgenest orphanage. Despite the fact that the children under Fraulein's Schwarz's thumb now received extra food, they did not thrive. In fact the average rate at which children in the two orphanages were growing was reversed.

FAITH AND HEALING

The importance of being part of a happy community is also demonstrated by studies on the impact of religious belief on health. It is well recognized, for example, that churchgoers are blessed with a longer life. A study sponsored by the US National Institute on Aging found that people who go to church regularly tend to be mentally and physically healthier than those who don't, and a recent review of 212 studies found that being religious is of particular benefit to alcoholics, addicts and the mentally ill.

I don't think it's desperately surprising that being part of a community and believing in a higher power can play a role in keeping you well. If healing is another way of saying that compassion and trust are vital components in the effectiveness of any medicine, who could argue with that? But self-proclaimed healers insist there's more to it. They believe they can tap into a mystical energy source, an extra force, something which is over and above the benefits to be derived from belief.

I have met many down-to-earth sensible people who say they have been cured of illnesses by healers despite being deeply sceptical about it all beforehand. David, a former policeman, for example, had been struggling along for years with a bad knee. He'd had three unsuccessful operations before he decided to give healing a go. It couldn't have been simpler. The healer spent a couple of minutes just allowing her hands to hover above his bad knee. After a few sessions of this David felt so much better that he took himself off to the golf course and has not looked back.

Then there's Mary, who started bleeding heavily from her vagina. She had an ultrasound scan which suggested she had fibroids – benign tumours in the muscle wall of the womb. A scan taken after five months of healing, however, showed that the fibroids had gone.

Her GP, Dr Michelle Langdon, who is also a healer, is not surprised by this. She believes that power transmitted through a healer's hands really can shrink a smooth muscle tumour or mend broken bones. So what does she think is going on? 'You scan your hand over these areas and you detect a blockage. When that blockage has cleared itself by the influx of energy, the whole system somehow is able to cope with the illness.'

Dr Langdon says the energy is coming through but not from her. So what is the evidence for the existence of this mysterious force? Well, in 1990 forty-four volunteers took part in a healing experiment.[5] The volunteers were all deliberately wounded with a precisely measured cut made on their forearms. They were then randomly allocated either to treatment from a healer or no treatment. To get round the problem of the placebo effect, it was important that none of the patients knew if they were being healed or not. So they constructed a room which had a small hole in the wall and the volunteers had to stick their injured arms through the hole. In half the cases these volunteers were waving their arms in an empty room, while the other twenty-two received no-touch healing; the healer sat quietly nearby, moving their hands over the limb without actually touching it. They found that after sixteen days the wounds of the unhealed group were still open, whereas the wounds of the healed group were almost completely recovered. Remarkable!

Unfortunately, when they repeated the experiment in 1996 with tighter controls there was no difference between the two groups. A team at Exeter University who study complementary medicine are now planning to do a variant of the experiment, this time using a one-way mirror to conceal either a healer or empty space.

A more convincing study comes from the *Southern Medical Journal*.[6] Patients going into San Francisco General Hospital coronary care unit were asked if they minded being prayed for by a group of 'born again' Christians; 393 patients agreed, fifty-seven refused.

A computer then decided which patients would be prayed for and which would not. Neither the patients nor the doctors were told. Not even the Christians doing the praying really knew who they were praying for; they were told the patient's first name, what they were in for and how they were doing. Essentially they prayed that the patients on their list would make a rapid recovery.

At the end of the study they broke open the secret codes and checked what had happened. What they found was that being prayed for made no difference to the number of days the patients spent in hospital or the amount of drugs they had to take when they were discharged from hospital. But it did make some difference: the group being prayed for were less likely to develop pneumonia, needed fewer antibiotics and were less likely to have had a heart attack while in intensive care.

The overall effect wasn't huge, but it was statistically significant: 85 per cent of patients being prayed for got better (163 out of 192), compared to 73 per cent of those who were not prayed for. Although the group being prayed for had been chosen randomly, the researchers double-checked that the computer hadn't, by chance, allocated healthier people to the prayer group in the first place. It hadn't.

I find it surprising there was an effect at all, but to put the size of this effect into perspective you might like to know that having a view is a rather more powerful aid to recovery. In a study published in *Science*, patients undergoing cholecystectomy (removal of the gallbladder) in a hospital were left to recover on one of two floors. The patients' rooms either looked out on to a brick wall or had a view with trees. The patients who could see the trees spent one day less in hospital and needed less than half of the number of painkilling injections.[7]

The critics of both studies will say, 'They're one-offs and one-off studies don't prove anything'. Believers will say the praying study was an artificial situation and we shouldn't be testing God in this way. Scientists will say, 'Give us a grant and we'll do more research and really sort this one out'.

I understand how having a view can lift your mood and aid recovery, but not how healing can work through unseen energy. If you do decide to put yourself in the hands of a healer, make sure it's through a reputable organization. I met a woman recently – I'll call her Daphne – who had been to a healer with a bad back. The healer told Daphne that she had not only been able to mend her back but had also sensed that Daphne's mother was ill and would die unless she was prayed for by the healer. Daphne handed over more than £5,000 to keep her mother from dying of a non-existent disease.

So, I end on the same note I began with: stay alert, be sceptical, ask awkward questions – and don't have blind trust in anyone. Trust me … I'm a doctor.

FURTHER INFORMATION

The Homeopathic Society
2 Powis Place
London WC1N 3HT
(0171) 837 9469

The Royal London Homeopathic Hospital
Great Ormond St
London WC1N 3HR
0171 837 8833

To find a qualified acupuncturist contact:

The British Acupuncture Council
Park House
206–208 Latimer Road
London W10 6RE
0181 964 0222

For information on finding a reputable healer send an SAE to:

National Federation of Spiritual Healers
Old Manor Farm, Church St
Sunbury on Thames
Middlesex TW16 6RG.

Or you could send an SAE to:

Spiritualists' National Union – Healing Committee
36 Newmarket
Otley
West Yorkshire LS21 3AE
http://www.netmedia.co.uk/users/healers/

NOTES

Chapter 1

1 *British Medical Journal (BMJ)* 1998, vol. 317, pp. 1097, 1111
2 *Guy's Hospital Gazette*, 1936, vol L, p. 7
3 *BMJ*, 1993, vol. 306, pp. 691–2
4 *BMJ*, 1994, vol. 308, p. 1374
5 *BMJ*, 1997, vol. 314, p. 1619
6 *BMJ*, 1998, vol. 316, p. 193–5
7 *BMJ*, 1988, vol. 296, pp. 839–40
8 E. Wilkes 'The Quality of Life' in Doyle, D, ed., *Palliative Care – the management of far advanced illness*, Charles Press, 1984, pp. 9–19
9 *Lancet*, 1993, vol. 341, pp. 473–6
10 *BMJ*, 1996, vol. 313, pp. 724–6
11 *British Journal of General Practice*, 1998, vol. 48, 1998, pp. 1081–2
12 *Lancet*, 1996, vol. 348, pp. 922–5
13 *Lancet*, 1998, vol. 352, p. 785

Chapter 2

1 *BMJ*, 1997, vol. 314, pp. 1591–2
2 Dowling and Barrett, *Doctors in the Making – the experience of pre-registration house officers*, SANS publications, 1991
3 *Health Trends*, vol. 28 no. 2
4 *British Journal of Bone Surgery*, 1996, vol. 78B, p. 178
5 *BMJ*, 1994, vol. 309, pp. 1408–9
6 *BMJ*, 1991, vol. 302, pp. 626–7; *BMJ*, 1993, vol. 306, pp. 1578–9
7 *BMJ*, 1992, vol. 304, pp. 1347–51
8 *BMJ*, 1994, vol. 308, p. 275
9 *BMJ*, 1997, vol. 315, News
10 *BMJ*, 1998, vol. 316, pp. 1853–8
11 *BMJ*, 1994, vol. 309, Letters
12 *BMJ*, 1995, vol. 311, pp. 630–1
13 *Health Service Journal*, 22 February 1996, pp. 26–9
14 *Trust Me, I'm a Doctor*, 20 November 1996
15 *BMJ*, vol. 295, pp. 533–5

16 Isobel Allen, *Doctors and their Careers: A New Generation* (London: Policy Studies Institute, 1988)
17 *British Journal of Hospital Medicine,* 1992, vol. 47, pp. 452–64)
18 *The Morbidity and Mortality of the Medical Profession: a Literature Review and Suggestions for Future Research* (BMA, 1993)
19 *Trust Me, I'm a Doctor,* 11 December 1996
20 *Doctor Magazine,* 16 October 1997
21 *BMJ,* 1994, vol. 309, p. 132
22 *The Citadel,* 25 June 1998

Chapter 3
1 *BMJ,* 1998, vol. 316, pp. 1685–6
2 *BMJ,* 1998, vol. 316, pp. 1685–6
3 *Health Service Journal,* 27 August 1998, Features
4 *BMJ,* 1994, vol. 309, pp. 1640–5
5 *Health Service Journal,* 27 August 1998, Features
6 *Private Eye,* issue 793, 8 May 1992
7 *Private Eye,* issue 797, 3 July 1992
8 *Private Eye,* issue 804, 9 October 1992
9 *Health Service Journal,* 27 August 1998, Features
10 *Hospital Doctor,* 22 February 1996, Features

Chapter 4
1 Corpus Debate, Bristol Medical School, 26 November 1998
2 *Cleft Palate Craniofacial Journal,* vol. 29, pp. 393–418
3 *Trust Me, I'm a Doctor,* 3 November 1997
4 *Private Eye,* issue 937, 14 November 1997
5 *BMJ,* 1992, vol. 290, pp. 345–7)
6 *Private Eye,* issues 957, 958, 960 August–September 1998
7 *Trust Me, I'm a Doctor,* 26 February 1999
8 Charles Vincent, ed., *Clinical Risk Management* (BMJ Books, 1995)
9 *The Relationship Between Hospital Volume and Health Care Outcomes,* CRD Report 8 (NHS Centre for Reviews and Dissemination, 1997)
10 *BMJ,* 1996, vol. 312, pp. 145–8
11 *Trust Me, I'm a Doctor,* 13 November 1996
12 *Hospital Doctor,* 17 September 1998, Features
13 *Lancet,* 1996, vol. 342, pp. 395–8
14 *BMJ,* 1997, vol. 314, pp. 1151–9
15 *Trust Me, I'm a Doctor,* 13 November 1996

16 'Patient Choice in Managing Cancer', *Drugs and Therapeutics Bulletin*, 1993, vol. 31, no. 20
17 *Trust Me, I'm a Doctor*, 10 November 1997
18 *BMJ*, vol. 306, pp. 732–3
19 *Trust Me, I'm a Doctor*, 10 March 1998
20 *BMJ*, 1998, vol. 317, p. 811

Chapter 5
1 *Lancet*, 1954, vol. ii, p. 321
2 'The Powerful Placebo', *Journal of the American Medical Association*, 1955, vol. 159, no. 17, pp. 1602–6.
3 *Pain*, 1988, vol. 33, pp. 303–11
4 H. M. Spiro, *Doctors, Patients and Placebos* (Yale University Press, 1986)
5 *BMJ*, 1996, vol. 313, p. 1008
6 John Yates, *Private Eye, Heart and Hip* (F. T. Healthcare, 1996)
7 *New England Journal of Medicine*, 1959, vol. 260, pp. 1115–18
8 *BMJ*, 1996, vol. 312, p. 613
9 L. Covi and L. Park, 'Nonblind Placebo Trial', *Archives of General Psychiatry*, 1965, vol. 12, pp. 336–45
10 *Lancet*, 1985, vol. i, p. 344
11 *BMJ*, 1948, vol. ii, pp. 790–2
12 *Millbank Quarterly*, 1994, vol. 72, pp. 225–58
13 John Allen Paulos, *Innumeracy* (Penguin 1988)
14 *BMJ*, 1987, vol. 294, pp. 1200–2

Chapter 6
1 *British Journal of Cancer*, 1998, vol. 78(1), pp. 129–35
2 *Lancet*, 1997, vol. 349, p. 1776
3 *BMJ*, 1991, vol. 303, pp. 565–8; also, 'Alcohol and mortality: a review', *Journal of Clinical Epidemiology*, 1995, vol. 488, pp. 445–65
4 *BMJ*, 1997, vol. 314, p. 1159
5 *BMJ*, 1997, vol. 314, p. 1159
6 *BMJ*, 1998, vol. 317, pp. 505–10
7 *Quarterly Journal of Studies into Alcohol*, 1973, vol. 34, pp. 1195–201
8 *Quarterly Journal of Studies into Alcohol*, 1970, vol. 5, pp. 67–85
9 *International Journal of Epidemiology*, 1998, vol. 27(3), pp. 438–43
10 *The European Journal of Cancer Prevention*, 1998, vol. 7(3), pp. 207–13
11 *BMJ*, 1996, vol. 313, pp. 1362–6
12 *BMJ*, 1997, vol. 314, p. 1666

13 *BMJ*, 1997, vol. 314, p. 629
14 *Journal of the American Medical Association*, 1998, vol. 279, pp. 1659–61
15 *BMJ*, 1997, vol. 315, pp. 722–9
16 *Journal of the American Medical Association*, 1997, vol. 279, pp. 23–8
17 *New England Journal of Medicine*, 1997, vol. 337, pp. 1491–9
18 *BMJ*, 1998, vol. 316, pp. 1047–51
19 *European Journal of Clinical Nutrition*, 1997, vol. 51, pp. 116–22

Chapter 7

1 *Journal of the American Medical Association*, 1995, vol. 273, p. 1113)
2 *American Journal of Epidemiology*, 1997, vol. 146, pp. 618–26
3 *BMJ*, 1997, vol. 314, p. 629
4 *Thorax*, 1997, vol. 52, pp. 628–33
5 *New England Journal of Medicine*, 1996, vol. 334, pp. 1145–9
6 *Scandinavian Journal of Infectious Diseases*, 1994, vol. 26, no. 1, pp. 1–6
7 *BMJ*, 1997, vol. 314, p. 634
8 *Lancet*, 1997, vol. 349, p. 9067
9 *Journal of the National Cancer Institute*, 1998, vol. 90, pp. 440–6
10 *Geriatrics*, 1998, vol. 53 suppl 1:S31–4
11 *Biochim Biophys Acta*, 1998, vol. 1404(3), pp. 427–34
12 *Journal of the American Medical Association*, 1997, vol. 277, pp.1775–81
13 *Lancet*, 1997, vol. 349, p. 9049
14 *Lancet*, 1998, vol. 351, p. 9098
15 *Lancet*, 1998, vol. 351, p. 9115
16 *BMJ*, 1997, vol. 314, p. 387
17 *Journal of the American Medical Association*, 1998, vol. 279, pp. 440–4
18 *New England Journal of Medicine*, 1998, vol. 338, pp. 94–9
19 *BMJ*, 1997, vol. 315, pp. 1641–4
20 *American Journal of Epidemiology*, 1983, vol. 117, pp. 320–5
21 *Gerontologist*, 1982, vol. 6, pp. 513–8

Chapter 8

1 *British Journal of Obstetrics and Gynaecology*, 1988, vol. 95(9), pp. 933–4
2 *American Journal of Public Health*, 1995, vol. 85, pp. 494–503
3 *Contraception*, 1994, vol. 49, pp. 56–72
4 *Lancet*, 1998, vol. 352, pp. 428–33
5 Royal Statistical Society
6 *Lancet*, 1996, vol. 347, p. 9017
7 *American Journal of Gynaecology*, December 1991

8 *British Journal of Urology*, 1998, vol. 160(4), p. 1337
9 *Biological Trace Elements Research*, 1996, vol. 53(1–3), pp. 65–83
10 *British Journal of Urology*, 1998, vol. 82(1), pp. 76–80
11 *BMJ*, 1992, vol. 305, pp. 609–13
12 *Where to be Born? The Debate and the Evidence* (Oxford National Perinatal Epidemiology Unit, 2nd ed, 1994)
13 *European Journal of Obstetrics and Gynaecology and Reproductive Biology*, 1997, vol. 73, pp. 1–4
14 *BMJ*, 1990, vol. 301, pp. 9–12
15 *BMJ*, 1995, vol. 311, pp. 1336–9
16 *British Journal of Psychiatry*, 1982, vol. 140, pp. 111–17
17 *BMJ*, 1997, vol. 314, p. 932

Chapter 9
1 *BMJ*, 1998, vol. 316, pp. 1356–9
2 *Back Pain: Report of a CSAG Committee on Back Pain* (HMSO, 1994)
3 *Low back pain evidence review* (Royal College of General Practitioners, 1996)
4 *Journal of the American Medical Association*, 1997, vol. 277, pp. 1940–4
5 *Annals of Internal Medicine*, 1996, vol. 125, pp. 81–8
6 *Journal of the American Medical Association*, 1998, vol. 279, pp. 1962–7, 1999–2000
7 *Journal of Affective Disorders*, 1986, vol. 10, pp. 67–75
8 *BMJ*, 1997, vol. 314, p. 1811
9 *New England Journal of Medicine*, 1995, vol. 332, pp. 621–8
10 Department of Transport
11 *Lancet*, 1996, vol. 347, p. 1642
12 *European Journal of Clinical Pharmacology*, 1994, vol. 46, pp. 517–22

Chapter 10
1 *Lancet*, 1994, vol. 344, p. 1601
2 *Lancet*, 1997, vol. 350, pp. 834–43
3 *Anaesthesia*, 1997, vol. 52, pp. 658–61
4 *Lancet*, 1951, vol. I, pp. 1316–18
5 *Subtle Energies*, vol. 1, pp. 1–20
6 *Southern Medical Journal*, 1988, vol. 81, pp. 826–9
7 *Science*, 1983, vol. 224, p. 420

INDEX

abbreviations for patient types 39–40
abortion, selenium and 138
abuse
hospital staff 52
patients 39–43
accountability of doctors 6, 59, 62
ACE inhibitors for heart failure 95–6
Action for Victims of Medical Accidents 84
acupuncture 186, 192–5
AD-36 virus 184
Addicted Physicians Programme 38
Advanced Trauma Life Support Provider Certificate 31
AIDS 20
alcohol
abuse in doctors 17–18, 19, 37–9
life expectancy 113, 117–21
side effects 119
allergies 190
alveolar bone grafting 69
Alzheimer's disease, vitamin E and 134
American Medical Association vii
Ames, Professor Bruce 114
amniocentesis 81–3, 103, 155
anaesthesia, pain and 184
angina 92
animal fats 125–6, 155, 182
antibiotics and middle ear infections 97
antidepressants 176–7
anti-hypertensive drugs and stroke 98

anti-oestrogen drugs 94–5
antioxidants 128, 131
anxiety 175–80
in doctors 18
apprenticeships 29–30
Arkley, Catherine 72
arterial switch operation 57
arthritis, acupuncture 195
asbestos 131
Asher, Richard 188
Asians, discrimination against 7–9
aspirin
blood clots 124–5
colds 174
heart attacks 90, 95–6, 97–8
assessment process 20–1
Association for Improvements in Maternity Services 165
asthma
allergic 190
diet and 130
Atkinson, Richard 183–4
audit
amniocentesis 81
compulsory 49, 61–2, 63
ECT 77
hip replacements 80
lack of 34, 47, 54, 58, 69
prostate surgery 77–8
secret 50
Avon Health Authority 58
Axsain 186–7

back problems following epidurals 162
back ache 166–9

Bandolier vii, 98
Bath GP training scheme 25–6
BBC Bristol 60
Beck, Aaron 179
bed design 169
Beecher, Henry 89–90
behaviour
    doctors 39–43
    in medical school 5–6
    postgraduate 49–43
behavioural therapy for depression
    178–80
betacarotene 112, 128, 130, 134
Beta-Carotene and Retinol Efficacy
    Trial (CARET) 130–1
biliary atresia 71–3
birds, length of life 142
birth 157–63
birth companion 163
blood clots 124–5
    alcohol and 118
    from Pill 146–7
blood pressure
    anti-hypertensive drugs 98
    heart disease and 124
bogus doctors 35–7
Bolsin, Dr Steve 50, 53–4, 55, 60
Boneloc 81
Bottomley, Virginia 56–7
bowel cancer, coffee and 121
brain damage following
    amniocentesis 83
breach birth 158
bread pills 92
breast cancer 43, 73–4, 103
    from Pill 147–8
breast examinations 95
breast reduction 85–6
brewer's yeast 111

Bristol Royal Infirmary cardiac
    unit 23, 44–64
British Acupuncture Council 199
British Association for Behavioural
    and Cognitive Therapy 180
British Liver Trust 157
British Medical Association vii
bullying by senior staff 30
Bulstrode, Professor Chris 15,
    79–80, 87–8, 104

cadaver use 9–10
caesarean section 159
Calder, Dr Ian 120
calendar method of contraception
    150
Calman, Kenneth 74
calorie
    consumption 182
    restriction studies 142
Cambridge University Medical
    School 9
cancer 73–6
    coffee and 121
    communication about 12–13
    morphine and 184–5
    risk from Pill 147
    vitamin E and 134
    see also specific cancers
Capital prosthesis 80
capsaicin cream for pain 186–7
capsules vs tablets 92
carbohydrate intake 183
carcinogens 114
Cardiac Arrest 41
cardiac arrests 31–2
cardiac units, paediatric 23, 44–64
carotenoids 129
carrots 130

case-mix 48
Certificate of Completion of
    Specialist Training 30
cervical screening 98–9
Chalmers, Thomas 133
Charnley prosthesis 80, 81
Charter Marks 56
chemotherapy doses 49
chest pain 92
children, obesity and 182–3
chilli treatment for pain 186–7
Chinese men, sperm 140
chiropractors 168, 188
cholecystectomy, laparoscopic 15,
    198
cholestasis in pregnancy 156–7
cholesterol levels 112–13, 122–6,
    128
    coffee and 122
    -lowering drugs 123
    tests 98
cleft palate repair 66–9
Clifford, Dr Mike 122
clinical examinations 20–1
Clinical Standards Advisory Group
    68–9
clinical trials 93–6
co-codamol for pain 185
coffee 114, 121–2
    for colds 173–4
cognitive behavioural therapy for
    depression 164, 177, 179–80
colds, common 132, 171–5
colonic cancer 114
colorectal cancer 75–6
    coffee and 121
colour of tablets 92
communication skills 14
    teaching 93, 102

competence 34–5, 49
complaints
    from junior doctors 47
    from students 15–16
    see also whistle-blowing
complementary medicines 188–99
condoms 145
consent 25
consultant-led service 30–1
consultants
    attitudes to students 25
    firms 29
    skills 34
contraception 144–51
Copperfield, Dr Tony 41
coronary artery disease
    alcohol and 118
    bypass grafts 73, 96
    cholesterol and 123–4
coronary care, praying and 197–8
cosmetic surgery 85–6
cough medicines 170
coughs 170
curriculum in medical schools 12

deaths of babies 32, 44–63
defence mechanisms 114–15
dehydration from alcohol 120
delivery 157–63
Department of Health, Bristol
    cardiac unit and 56
depression 175–80
    in doctors 37
    following birth 163–4
Devlin, Brendan 78
Dhasmana, Mr 23, 54, 60, 62
DHEA 138, 142–3
Dhurandhar, Nikil 183–4
diabetic neuropathy pain 90, 186

diagnosis, communicating 12–14
diamorphine misuse 41
diarrhoea, nitrates and 116
diet 111–26, 133
    obesity and 182–3
dieting 181–4
dipterpenes 122
disciplinary procedures, GMC and
    8
discrimination
    against ethnic minorities 7
    against women 6–7, 18–19
dissection of human body 9–10
DNA damage 128
doctor
    bogus 35–7
    female consultant 7
    fund-holding 51
    –patient communication 12–13,
    100–7
    portrayal on TV 41–2
    questions to ask 105–7
    reasons for becoming 3–4
    referral to surgeons by 61
    whistle-blowing 28, 38
Doyle, Dr Peter 70–1, 72
Drabu, Khalid 79–80
drop-out rate 22
dummy see placebo
duodenal ulcer, pain relief 90

E. coli in food 116
ear infections, middle 97
Edinburgh Postnatal Depression
    Scale 163
egg consumption 112
elderly nursing 27–8
electroconvulsive therapy (ECT) 77
Elite prosthesis 81

emergency care 33, 34
    in private hospitals 84
emotional support for patients 93
empathy 14
endometrial cancer and Pill 148
endorphin release, placebos and 90
energy
    faith healing 196–7
    from oxygen 127
    lines 193
Entonox 161
epidural for delivery 161, 162
episiotomy 159
    repairs 28
equipment, need for training 33
Ericson technique 153
Ernst, Professor 194
Eskimos, fish in diet 125
Esmail, Dr Aneez 8
ethanol and hangovers 121
ethics
    body dissection 10
    placebos 93
    sex selection 152
ethnic minorities, discrimination
    against 7–9
Everington, Dr Sam 8
examinations
    intimate 40, 41
    in medical school 20–1
exercise 138–9
    and obesity 182–4
Exeter prosthesis 80, 81

faith
    healing 195–8
    in medicine 188
Family Planning Association
    150–1

fatigue 27
fat
    in diet 125–6
    levels in obesity 182
    animal, infertility and 155
feedback to health staff 102, 104
femoral fracture 15
fertility treatment 40
fetal monitoring 81–3, 158–9
fibrinogen levels, heart disease and 124
fibroids, faith healing 196
fish in diet 125
Fisher, Peter 190
fluoxetine for postnatal depression 164
folic acid 131, 134–6
food *see* diet
free radicals 128, 142
Freedom of Information Act 50
Freud, Sigmund 177
fruit and vegetables 112, 128–30
fund-holding 51

gallbladder removal 15
    recovery 198
Gardner, Dr Tony 46, 51
General Medical Council
    Bristol investigation 62, 63
    disciplinary procedures 8
Ghaly, Dr George 193
Goldenberg, Dr Joseph 111
grave robbing 9–10
grieving process for patients 13
Griffiths, Sir Roy 51
Guillebaud, Professor John 147
Guy's Hospital 46
    Christmas show 7–8
gynaecology 42–3

gynaecology *continued*
    behaviour of doctors 40
haemophilia, sex selection and 152
Hahnemann, Samuel 189–90
Hammersmith Hospital 45–6
hangovers 120
Hawkins, Catherine 61
hay fever 190
Heald, Bill 75
Health Address Book 96
Health Information First 165
heart attack
    aspirin and 90, 95–6, 97–8
    diet and 125
    sex and 141
    vitamin E and 134
heart disease
    alcohol and 113, 117–21
    cholesterol and 113, 122–6
    diet and 130
    folic acid and 134, 135
    vitamin C and 133
heart failure, ACE inhibitors and 95–6
Hemila, Professor 132
Hill, Mathew 60
Hill, Sally 82
hip replacements 29, 79–81, 104
Hislop, Ian 50
HIV, selenium deficiency and 137
home births 158–60
Homeopathic Society 198
homeopathy 189–92
homocysteine 135
Horton, Richard 43
hospital
    admissions 53
    births 158–60
    discharges 53

hospital *continued*
  pain relief in 184
  trust formation 51
hours, junior doctors 30
house jobs 22–5
house officers 22, 33
Huli people 140
human dissection 9–10
humour of doctors 18–20, 39–43, 46
hydrogen peroxide 128
hygiene and colds 175

iatrogenic risks in births 158
Iddon, Victoria 72
ileus 191
immune system, vitamin E and 134
impotence 153
  placebos and 90
in vitro fertilization 152
incompetence 42, 63, 86
incontinence following pregnancy 159
Indians, sperm 140
infections in hospital 160
infertility 153–5
  alcohol and 119–20
influenza, selenium and 137
information to patients 13, 100–2
inguinal hernia repair 33
Institute for Longevity Research 143
intensive care units in private hospitals 84
intubations 26, 32
itching in pregnancy 155–6
IUDs 145–6

James, Linda 74
jargon see language
jaundice in babies 71
Jauniaux, Eric 82
Jersey 27–8
Joiner, Dr Ian 38
junior doctors
  hours 30
  mistakes 30
  tiredness 27
  training 29–35
  whistle-blowing 28
Justins, Dr Douglas 184, 185

Kasai procedure 71–3
Kennedy, Professor Ian 58
keyhole surgery 94
knee pain, faith healing 196

labour wards 30
Lancet vii
Langdon, Dr Michelle 196–7
language
  in medical school 4–5, 10–11
  in public school 4
laparoscopic surgery 33
Law of Halves 163–4
learning on the job 22–43
Ledward, Rodney 23, 42, 65
Leibel, Rudolph 181
lettuce 116, 117
levornorgestrel 146
'like cures like' 190
liposuction 85
Lithuanians, cholesterol levels 123, 129
liver
  problems in pregnancy 156
  transplants 70–1

longevity 141–3
LST Clinic 86
lumbar punctures 161
lung cancer
    diet and 130, 131
    tea and 122
    vitamin C and 133
lycopene 129

mammary artery tying 92
masons 59
mastectomy, pain following 186
masturbation 141
maxillofacial surgery vs plastic
    surgery 69
McMaster, Professor Paul 70
media and food scares 113
Medical Devices Agency 80
medical revues 7–8, 20, 39
medical school 3–21
Mediterranean diets 126
Medline vii
Memon, Dr Mohammed Ashraf 8
mental illness 175–80
    in doctors 37, 164
mesorectal excision, total 75
meta-analysis 94
metabolic rate
    and life span 142
    and obesity 181
methanol and hangovers 121
micro-organisms, oxygen and 127
MIND 180
minimum dilutions 190
miscarriage following
    amniocentesis 83
mistakes
    junior doctors 27–8
    students 16–17

mitral valvuloplasties 62
Monica study 123, 135–6
Morice, Dr Alan 170
morning sickness 194
morphine 184–5
Muirhead-Allwood, Sarah 79
multiple choice questions 20

naproxen for pain 185
National Back Pain Association 169
National Federation of Spiritual
    Healers 199
National Institutes on Aging 143
nausea, acupuncture for 193, 194
negative automatic thoughts 179
neurotic symptoms, placebos 93
New England Journal of Medicine
    vii
NHS
    crises 52
    finances 68
    management 51, 52
    reforms 52
    staff abuse 52
nitrates 113, 115–16
Norman, Mike 35
Number Needed to Harm 107
Number Needed to Screen 107
Number Needed to Treat 97–8, 107
nurses
    portrayal on TV 42
    teaching doctors 15, 23, 25, 26
    whistle-blowing 15
nutrition see diet

O'Donnell, Michael 58
O'Reagan, Paddy 4
obesity 190–4
obstetric cholestasis 156–7

Obstetric Cholestasis Information and Support Service 157
obstetrics 28, 31
oesophageal cancer, tea and 122
oestrogen, sperm counts and 155
olive oil 125–6
opium 191
oral contraceptive pill 146–8
orgasm and death 139–41
osteoarthritis for pain 186
osteopaths 168, 188
ovarian cancer and Pill 148
oxidants 128
oxygen toxicity 127, 142

P6 point 193, 194
paediatrics 25–7
  cardiac unit 23, 44–64
  resuscitation training 32
pain 184–7
  acupuncture 194
  neck 166–9
  relief in birth 161–2
Pain Society 187
painkillers 90–1
Panorama 61
paracetamol
  colds 174
  pain 185
  toxicity 114–15
Parnell, Diane and Terry 83
pathology 9–10, 16–17
patient–doctor communication 12–13, 100–7
patients
  abuse 39–43
  ignorance of surgery 11
  information to 73
  notes 40

Patients' Association 96
Pauling, Linus 132, 172
Pavlov, Ivan 178
Pawade, Ash 64, 103–4
pay 28
pellagra 111–12
pelvic floor exercises 159–60
pelvic inflammatory disease
  from IUDs 145–6
  and Pill 148
perineal damage in birth 159
Personna 148–9
pesticides 114
pethidine 162
phobias 178
physicians see doctors
Physicians' Health Study 130
Pinehill Hospital 85
pituitary gland, alcohol and 120
placebos 88–93, 164
plastic surgery vs maxillofacial surgery 69
Poles, heart disease and 126, 129
polyunsaturated fats 125–6
postoperative ileus 191
poverty 96
power struggles 52
praise to health staff 102
pravastatin 97
praying 196–7
pregnancy 151–7
  contraception against 144–51
  ectopic, from IUDs 146
  folic acid and 134–6
  by oral route 144
  unplanned 145
premenstrual tension, vitamin B_6 and 136–7
Private Eye 50–1, 54, 56–7

private medicine 83–6
prostate cancer
    screening 98
    vitamin E and 134
    surgery 77–8
prostheses, hip 79–81, 104
Prozac 163, 176–7
psychotherapy 177, 178–80
ptosis 62
public school environment 4–6
pyridoxine 136–7

quality
    control in hospitals 86
    of NHS service 51

racial discrimination 7–9
radionics 188–9
randomized controlled trials 93–6
rare operations 66–73
ratamorphic fallacy 113–14
Rayman, Dr Margaret 137–8
reassurance to patient 101
rectal surgery 75–6
referrals 61
Reilly, Dr David 190
religion and healing 196
Research Council for
    Complementary Medicine 193
reserpine, impotence and 90
resuscitation 31–2
    in private hospitals 84
retinol 130–1
rhythm method 148–9
Rice-Evans, Cathy 131–2
risk
    management 73
    stratification 48–9, 70
Royal Brompton Hospital 46

Royal College of Obstetricians
    and Gynaecologists guidelines
    82
Royal College of Surgeons 68
Royal London Homeopathic
    Hospital 199
Roylance, John 56
rusting 127

Saed, Dr Mohammed 36–7
St Bartholomew's Hospital 8
St John's Comprehensive School,
    Marlborough 4
St Thomas's Medical School 5, 6,
    11, 23
saliva 116
salt water for colds 174
Sanders, Roy 69
screening tests 98–9
second opinions 102
secondary taste cortex 183–4
secrecy 6, 12–13, 49–50
selective serotonin re-uptake
    inhibitors 176–7
selenium 128, 137–8
    infertility and 154
self-assessment 49
self-regulation 23
sex and death 139–41
sex selection in pregnancy 151–3
sexual dissatisfaction 141
sexual drive, Prozac and 177
sham acupuncture 193–4
sham surgery 92, 94
Shaw, Professor William 67
shoulder dystocia 31
sigmoidoscopies 41
Sikora, Professor Karol 74–5
Smith, Dr Andrew 173–4

smoking
    acupuncture for 193–4
    heart disease and 124
    infertility and 153
    lung cancer 131
    oxidants and 128
social discrimination 7
Society of Cardiothoracic Surgeons 49
special care baby units 25
specialists vs non-specialists 66–73, 103–4
sperm
    characteristics 151–3
    counts 94–5, 154–5
    dyeing 153
    infertility and 153
    motility 138
    retention 140
spina bifida 131, 134–6
spinal cord compression 168
Spiritualists' National Union 199
Squier, Waney 83
Stanmoor prosthesis 80, 81
starch intake 183
starvation, living longer and 141–3
statins 123
Stirrat, Professor Gordon 65
stomach cancer 115
Stopes, Marie 144, 150
streptokinase for heart attacks 97–8
streptomycin trials for TB 94
stress in doctors 17–18, 24, 37–9
stroke 76–7
    anti-hypertensive drugs and 98
    diet and 129
    folic and 135
    vitamin C and 133
Struck Off and Die 46, 59

students
    mistakes 16–17
    whistle-blowing 15–16, 26
Summerland, Professor Brian 68
supervision, lack 33
support groups 96
surgeons
    attitudes to students 24
    bogus 35–7
    female consultant 7
    nicknames 23
    struck off 23
surgery
    records 69
    success rate quotes 54
Sweetnam, Sir Rodney 43
sympto-thermal method of contraception 149–50

tablets
    colour 92
    placebo 89
Taylor, Bob 103
tea 121–2
teacher training 21
television watching 182
thalidomide 194
three wise men system 38, 55
thrombo-embolism from Pill 146–7
tiredness 27
tomato sauce 129
training
    communication skills 14, 93, 102
    courses for surgeons 15
    inadequacy 20–1, 28–35
    junior doctors 29–35
    in medical school 11–12

training *continued*
    schemes 25–6
    structured 30–1
transcutaneous electrical nerve
    stimulation for pain 186
Treasure, Tom 48
tricyclic antidepressants 176
trust, misplaced 36
tubercular meningitis, depressive
    signs and 177
tuberculosis, streptomycin trials 94
twins
    birth 158
    exercise studies 138–9

UK Council for Psychotherapy 180
ultrasound amniocentesis 81–3

Vallance-Owen, Dr Andrew 84
vegetables and fruit 112, 128–30
Vickers, Dr Andrew 193
viruses
    cold 171
    selenium and 137
vitamins 130–6
    supplements 131–8
    vitamin A 128, 154
    vitamin B 111
    vitamin B_6 136–7
    vitamin B_{12} 133
    vitamin C 128, 131–3, 154, 172
    vitamin E 113, 128, 131–2,
        133–4, 154

Waddell, Professor Gordon 166–7
waiting lists 29–30
Wald, Professor Nick 135
Walker, Duncan 64
walking 138–9, 183

water birth 160
water intake 183
Webb, Beverley 85
well-being 195
West One Clinic 86
whistle-blowing 15–17, 26, 28, 38,
    43
    Bristol cardiac unit 44–64
White, Simon 66–7
William Harvey Hospital 42
Williams, John 69
wine 118
Wisheart, James 45, 50, 54–5,
    57–63
Wolpert, Professor Lewis 176
women
    abuse against 40
    discrimination against 6–7, 19
workaholism 39
wound healing 116, 197
Wrede, David 31

X-ray, spinal 167

Yuzpe contraceptive method 146

zinc for colds 172–3